Clinical Communication Skills in Medicine

This book takes readers through 45 challenging scenarios to teach communication skills in medicine. It follows the revised format of the Practical Assessment of Clinical Examination Skills (PACES) exam conducted by the Royal College of Physicians in the UK, which tests communication skills twice in two separate stations. As most scenarios in this book have been created in an acute medical unit setting, the approach followed should also appeal to senior medical students and trainees in internal medicine and general practice at all levels. Readers will learn:

- How to convey abnormal test results and break bad news
- How to discuss the diagnosis of a chronic disease and negotiate a management plan
- How to communicate with patients who pose an ethical dilemma
- How to communicate with challenging patients and relatives
- What to tell patients or relatives when things go wrong
- How to communicate with patients and relatives regarding end-of-life issues

Key Features:

- Takes readers through a simple, step-by-step approach to skilfully dealing with common challenging communication scenarios they face in their daily practice
- Guides readers on how to communicate in layman's terms without using medical jargon, as it is fully dialogued, proving particularly helpful to non-UK candidates whose first language is not English
- Simplifies several complex ethical and medicolegal principles, such as treatment of patients lacking capacity, dealing with patients who refuse consent, confidentiality, counselling a non-compliant patient, basic genetic counselling, management of patients who demand non-indicated investigations or treatments, open disclosure after a medical error, preparing an advance decision and lasting power of attorney, issues around brain death and organ donation, tube feeding, 'Do Not Attempt Resuscitation' (DNAR) orders, and referral to the coroner.

MasterPass Series

The Final FRCA Constructed Response Questions
A Practical Study Guide, 2E
Elizabeth Combeer, Mitul Patel

Diagnostic EMQs
A Comprehensive Collection for Medical Examinations
Syed Hussain, Umber Rind, Jawed Noori, Yasmean Kalam, Haseeb Ata, Emanuel Papageorgiou

Passing the Final FFICM
High-Yield Facts for the MCQ & OSCE Exams
Muzzammil Ali

Cases in Haematology
For the MLA and PLAB
Aaron Niblock

Postgraduate Ophthalmology Exam Success
Maneck Nicholson, Anjali Nicholson, Syed Faraaz Hussain

Pass the MRCP (SCE) Neurology Revision Guide
Dhananjay Gupta

Advanced ENT MCQs
Training to Pass the FRCS (ORL-HNS) Part 1
Peter Kullar, Jameel Muzaffar, Joseph Manjaly

Clinical Communication Skills in Medicine
A Primer for MRCP PACES
Ernest Suresh

For more information on this series, please visit
https://www.routledge.com/MasterPass/book-series/CRCMASPASS

Clinical Communication Skills in Medicine

A Primer for MRCP PACES

Ernest Suresh MD, FRCP (London)

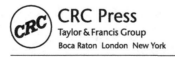

CRC Press
Taylor & Francis Group
Boca Raton London New York

CRC Press is an imprint of the
Taylor & Francis Group, an **informa** business

First edition published 2025
by CRC Press
2385 NW Executive Center Drive, Suite 320, Boca Raton FL 33431

and by CRC Press
4 Park Square, Milton Park, Abingdon, Oxon, OX14 4RN

CRC Press is an imprint of Taylor & Francis Group, LLC

© 2025 Ernest Suresh

ISBN: 978-1-032-87567-5
ISBN: 978-1-032-87566-8
ISBN: 978-1-003-53333-7

DOI: 10.1201/9781003533337

Typeset in Sabon
by Apex CoVantage, LLC

Contents

SECTION III
Capacity, Consent, and Confidentiality

SECTION IV
Challenging Patients and Relatives

SECTION V
When Things Go Wrong

SECTION VI
End-of-Life Issues

Preface

This book takes you through 45 challenging cases in medicine to help you hone your skills in communicating with patients or relatives and to understand the key ethical principles. Although it is primarily targeted at those sitting for MRCP PACES, it should also appeal to senior undergraduate medical students and trainees in internal medicine and general practice at all levels.

In the two 'communication' stations, examiners will test four different skills, including (1) clinical communication, (2) managing patients' concerns, (3) clinical judgement, and (4) maintaining patient welfare. The scenarios are chosen to test your skills in (1) conveying an abnormal test result or breaking bad news, (2) counselling about a disease or negotiating a management plan, (3) handling consent- and confidentiality-related issues, (4) communicating with challenging patients or relatives, (5) dealing with medical error, and (6) discussing end-of-life issues. The scenarios are carefully vetted by the College to ensure that you can complete the task in ten minutes. On the day of the exam, the two examiners will calibrate each scenario and agree on what should constitute a satisfactory performance for each skill.

You will be given five minutes to read the scenario before entering the room. I can't emphasise enough how important it is to **read the details of the case very carefully** during that time. You will receive an unsatisfactory mark if you give incorrect information to the patient (e.g. If you say '*Your cancer has spread throughout your belly*' when the scenario states that 'the scan reported liver metastases'). It is also important to clearly understand what you are being asked to do. Consider the following example: the candidate's task is to convey the diagnosis of tuberculosis to an anxious patient who was recently investigated extensively for her weight loss and to discuss the next steps.

CANDIDATE *(who did not read the scenario properly):*   I understand that you were recently diagnosed with tuberculosis. I am here to discuss the treatment.

PATIENT *(who is shocked):*   What! I have been here for a week, and no one told me that I had tuberculosis!

You can imagine how difficult it will be to get out of this mess. You will be spending the first few minutes trying to calm her down and apologising for the oversight, thus unnecessarily losing some valuable time. You may not have enough time left at the end to talk about important issues, like isolation or testing for HIV, resulting in an unsatisfactory mark for clinical communication, managing patients' concerns, and clinical judgement (and possibly a borderline for maintaining patient welfare).

You cannot (and should not) plan the entire conversation before you enter the station, as it will largely depend on what the patient tells you, but it is a good idea to **write down the** *important points that you need to convey*. Think what the examiners might have put down on their calibration sheet for you to get a satisfactory mark for each skill. I have summarised these points at the end of each case. You should also *think of some questions that the patient is likely to ask you*, which are not difficult to anticipate (e.g. '*How long do you think I will live?*' [advanced cancer], '*Can you not tell my partner?*' [new diagnosis of HIV], '*Are my children at risk of getting this condition?*' [Huntington's disease]). You are allowed to refer to your notes, but I would discourage the habit of writing when the patient is talking to you.

After you enter the station, do not forget to *greet the examiners and the patient*. Always *introduce yourself* and *confirm the identity of the patient* (or relationship to the patient if you are talking to a relative). In PACES, you won't be sent into the wrong station, but you must still demonstrate it to the examiners! Thereafter, try not to be conscious of their presence, although it is difficult to be natural when you are being watched. If the patient is angry, remain calm and composed. Let it not unnerve you. Unlike in real life, the actors will be told that you only have ten minutes, so they will calm down if you say something reassuring (e.g. '*I can see that you are upset. I will try my best to explain.*').

Remember to *tell the patient about the purpose of the consultation* at the start. For most scenarios, you must *start with an open-ended question*. Do not interrupt soon after asking the open-ended question, unless the patient is going off-track, which is unlikely in PACES. Always *ask what they have been told already*. During the course of the conversation, you should *elicit their ideas, concerns, and expectations* (ICE), which will give you an idea of what is important to them. One patient with tension headache may tell you that he came to consult you because his '*wife was nagging [him] to see a doctor*', while another may tell you that his '*aunt suffered with a similar headache and she was diagnosed with a brain tumour*'. Clearly, these two patients need to be counselled differently.

For some scenarios (e.g. conveying critical or abnormal test results), *ask the patient if it is a good time to talk* ('*I have the results of your scan. Is this a good time to talk?*'). This question may seem ludicrous in PACES (the actor is not going to ask you to come after some time!), but it is, again, to demonstrate to the examiners that you understand the importance of talking to the patient or the relative at the right time. However, do not follow a rigid approach and ask this question as a standard. There is obviously no need for this question if the patient has come to consult you in the outpatient clinic or they have already told you, '*I can't wait to find out the results of my tests*'. Once you have told the patient that you have the results of the tests, do not spend too much time on questions like '*How much do you want to know?*' or '*Would you like to have anyone else with you?*' Keep it brief. It is very annoying to watch when this is dragged for too long, especially when you do this to an anxious patient who is worried about cancer. Another approach is to break the bad news first, give some time for the patient to digest it, and then ask if they would like you to go over in detail or only hear the bare minimum.

When you break bad news, always *give a warning shot* and follow it with a *momentary pause*. Deliver the information in *small chunks*, and *pause at regular intervals to check their understanding* ('*Are you with me so far? Would you like me to go over anything again?*'). Do not talk faster than the rate at which the patient can process the information. Allow *moments of silence* if you have delivered bad news. You must *avoid jargon* at all costs. Repeated use of jargon is one of the easiest ways to fail this station. *Do not overload the patient with too much information*, especially if the patient is in an emotional state. However, in the exam setting, the actor will be trained to recover quickly, and you must manage to somehow convey the key points that the examiners might have put down on their calibration sheets. If you think it will enhance understanding, do not hesitate to *draw illustrative diagrams* to explain.

You should pitch the *conversation to the education level of the patient* (e.g. '*You have a blood clot in your brain*' instead of '*I suspect you have had a stroke, which is caused by a blood clot blocking the blood vessel that supplies a part of your brain*'). You can ask the patient to stop you if you are going too fast. Your *English doesn't have to be perfect*. English is not the first language for most candidates who sit the PACES (and for many examiners too!). PACES is taken by candidates around the world, and examiners realise that you will be talking in your own language in the country where you practice. You will still get a satisfactory mark as long as you help the patient understand what you said.

Your *conversation must be patient-centred*. It should be a dialogue, not a monologue. Listen to the patient; don't just hear (there is a difference). When you discuss the treatment, present the choices and *enable the patient to make an informed decision. Do not adopt a paternalistic attitude*. For example, if you are recommending prophylactic treatment to a patient with gout, you should say, '*I would recommend a tablet called allopurinol to reduce the uric acid level and prevent the gout attacks*', not '*You must take allopurinol because you are getting frequent attacks of gout*'. For patients with chronic disease, you should *negotiate a management plan* that suits the patient and not offer generic advice. Try to convey hope and optimism, but *do not give false reassurances* just to get out of an uncomfortable situation (e.g. '*You will be OK, don't worry*' to a patient with terminal cancer).

Once you have delivered the bad news, *respond appropriately to the patient's emotions*. Say something reassuring (e.g. '*I wish things were different*', '*I am sorry that the scan result didn't turn out as well as we would have liked*', '*I understand how difficult this must be for you*'). Although not usually marked as a criterion for satisfactory performance, *non-verbal communication is as important as verbal*. Soft skills like body language, responding to non-verbal cues, and showing empathy will surely give an overall good impression. Do not have a flat affect or talk in a monotonous voice. Do not hesitate to *apologise if a mistake has been committed*, but do not repeat this several times. Most importantly, the sorry must come from your heart and not just the lips. How you say it is more important than what you say!

As the new format has removed the five-minute interaction with the examiner, your *clinical judgement* will be tested during your ten-minute interaction with the patient (e.g. ethical issues, organ donation, referral to the coroner, issues around 'do not attempt resuscitation' order, tube feeding, complaints process, genetic counselling). If a patient wishes to discharge himself against medical advice, testing his capacity and then allowing him to go home with appropriate advice will demonstrate to the examiners that you are aware that autonomy takes precedence over beneficence in an adult with mental capacity. Do not forget to *advise a patient to stop driving* for certain medical conditions (e.g. diabetes on insulin, cardiac syncope, seizures, sleep apnoea, transient ischaemic attack, acute coronary syndrome, visual loss). There is no need to remember the exact duration for which they must stop driving (you can tell them that you will check online). You will get points as long as you remember to ask the patient to stop driving. For patients with occupational lung disease, do not forget to *advise the patient regarding compensation*.

In the communication encounters, you may be given an *unsatisfactory mark for maintaining patient welfare if you hurt the patient emotionally*. Consider the following example:

PATIENT:	Could this be cancer, Doctor?
CANDIDATE:	Yes, it's possible. We'll get a CT scan of your chest and tummy, mammogram, camera tests, and so forth.
PATIENT *(looking really concerned)*:	How soon can you . . .?

CANDIDATE INTERRUPTS HER	I forgot to ask you one question earlier. Do you live in a
(while looking down on his sheet of paper):	bungalow or a house?
PATIENT:	I live in a bungalow. Why are you asking?
CANDIDATE:	That's good. You don't have to climb stairs with all your pain, then.

It clearly conveys insensitiveness and lack of concern. Rather than talking in a reassuring manner, the candidate was fixed on getting through the list of questions that he had written before entering the station. Not being *tactful while asking for sensitive information* is another reason for failing this skill. If you must obtain a sexual history, always start with '*I hope you won't mind if I ask you some sensitive questions, as it will help me find out what is wrong*'.

At the end, leave at least a minute to *summarise the main points* in a clear and concise manner. It should not be a repetition of the points that you already mentioned but, rather, a *plan for moving forward*. Use this time to go over what you and the patient agreed, discuss the next steps or follow-up arrangements, tell them that you will give them time to think through the issues that you discussed (if you were not able to reach an agreement), provide advice on troubleshooting issues, or offer to give some written information or details of useful websites. You can also tell them that you will write down the main points on a piece of paper and give it to them later so that they won't forget what you discussed. Do not feel disappointed if you did not manage to convince a patient. It only reflects what happens in real life and will not result in an unsatisfactory mark. The examiners only want to see how you conducted the consultation overall (e.g. giving clear advice for troubleshooting issues for a patient who wishes to leave the hospital against medical advice). Do not continue talking until the last second. Leave the last ten seconds free, as you'll have to go and examine the respiratory system or abdomen as soon as the bell rings!

No book can cover all possible scenarios, but you can follow the same approach or principles for related scenarios (e.g. 'missed stroke' [case 30] for any patient in whom the diagnosis is delayed, 'type 1 diabetes' [case 2] for any young patient diagnosed with a chronic disease, 'Huntington's disease' [case 22] for patients diagnosed with a genetic condition). I have given examples of case variations for several cases. There are several other challenging aspects of communication that we all face in real life (e.g. cross-cultural communication, communicating with people with low literacy), but they are beyond the scope of this book (and the PACES exam). I hope you will apply the knowledge gained from this book even after passing PACES and continue to improve this skill throughout your career.

About the Author

Dr Suresh is currently the head of medicine at Ng Teng Fong General Hospital in Singapore. Over the last three decades, he has worked in three different countries with contrasting healthcare systems and cultures. He has been teaching MRCP candidates for over two decades and has received more than a dozen teaching excellence awards in the last ten years alone. He has regularly published educational review articles on a wide range of topics in peer-reviewed internal medicine journals and has written an acute medicine handbook to guide the junior doctors in his hospital. His previous book, *Clinical Consultation Skills in Medicine: A Primer for MRCP PACES*, takes readers through a simple, clear, and rational approach to 63 common presenting symptoms or laboratory abnormalities in medicine.

He believes that all doctors, regardless of their speciality, should practice holistically and learn to treat the person that has the illness and not just the illness the person has. He considers himself an 'old-fashioned clinician' and pays a lot of attention to bedside clinical skills and communication, the essential traits that the Royal College expects PACES candidates to possess.

Section 1

Conveying Abnormal Test Results

The 51-Year-Old Woman with a Possible Brain Tumour

This 51-year-old secondary school teacher was admitted to the acute medical unit (AMU) earlier today after a brief episode of shaking of the left upper limb and unresponsiveness at home. The episode was witnessed by her husband. She reported no similar episodes in the past and was previously in good health. She was not taking any regular medication and did not smoke, drink alcohol, or use illicit drugs. She was not aware of anyone in her immediate family with epilepsy.

Physical examination at the time of admission was unremarkable. Her vital signs were normal, and Glasgow Coma Scale was 15. There were no focal neurological deficits. The admitting doctor diagnosed focal seizures and arranged some investigations. He did not tell her much except that he would arrange a brain scan and some blood tests.

Her full blood count, blood glucose, liver, renal and thyroid function, serum calcium, phosphate and magnesium, chest X-ray, and 12-lead electrocardiogram are all normal. However, the non-contrast computed tomography (CT) scan of her brain has been reported as showing 'a 3 cm lesion in the right frontal lobe, which is highly suspicious of a growth'. The radiologist has recommended further evaluation with a contrast magnetic resonance imaging (MRI) scan.

You are the medical registrar in the AMU. Your task is to discuss the results of her tests and the next steps with her.

- Introduce yourself and confirm her identity. Tell her that you have come to discuss her test results.
- Find out what happened, and ask what she has been told so far.

There is no need to obtain a detailed history. You should mainly use the time to (1) explain the diagnosis of focal seizures, (2) let her know the results of the CT scan and the next steps, (3) provide some general advice, and (4) answer any questions that she might have.

She says she feels well. She has no recollection of what happened that morning and only found out from her husband later. He told her that he first noticed some twitching of the fingers of her left hand, which rapidly moved up the arm, and she was soon shaking the entire limb. She was unresponsive at that time, and her head and eyes were turned to the right side. The shaking only lasted a couple of minutes, but she was drowsy and confused for several minutes after the episode. She has never experienced something like this before. The doctor who saw her earlier only told her that he would arrange a brain scan and some blood tests. She is anxious to find out why this happened and what the tests showed.

Seizures are broadly classified as focal and generalised. *Focal seizures* begin on one side of the brain, while *generalised seizures* begin on both sides simultaneously. Focal seizures are classified as *focal aware* or *focal impaired awareness* depending on whether or not they affect awareness. Loss of awareness in focal seizures occurs when the seizure activity involves the reticular activating system. Generalised seizures, by comparison, always affect awareness.

Her description suggests focal seizures (as the seizure activity involved only one limb) with impaired awareness (as she was unresponsive at that time and has no recollection of the event). Her husband's description of the ictal phase suggests Jacksonian march, which occurs due to the seizure activity spreading along the motor cortex.

There may be an underlying cause for the seizure (e.g. brain tumour, encephalitis, intracranial haemorrhage, hypoglycaemia, alcohol withdrawal) and a trigger (e.g. sleep deprivation, flashing lights). Some patients may experience an aura before the ictal phase, depending on where the seizure activity originates (e.g. visual hallucinations, unusual smell or taste, feeling of *déjà vu*, nausea, rising sensation in the epigastrium). The post-ictal phase occurs in generalised and focal impaired awareness seizure. It may manifest as lethargy, confusion, drowsiness, or Todd's paralysis.

- Tell her that *the episode was most likely caused by a seizure*.

'That must have been frightening. I am glad to hear that you are feeling well now. Let me explain why this happened. If there is anything that you don't understand, please feel free to stop me. [Momentary pause.] Based on your description, I suspect the shaking of your limb was caused by fits.'

She says she once witnessed one of her students having fits. He was stiff all over and shaking all four limbs at that time. She asks if you are sure she had fits, as her husband told her that she was shaking only one limb.

- Tell her that *seizures may be generalised or focal*.

'Fits occur because of excessive firing of signals by the brain cells. If both the right and left sides of the brain fire excessively at the same time, it causes all four limbs to shake and makes the person unconscious. If only a small area on one side of the brain fires, it causes just one limb to shake. We call this focal fits. Focal fits can sometimes make a person unconscious. It happens when the firing spreads to involve the parts of the brain that keep us awake. Your husband's account is in keeping with focal fits.'

After checking if she understood what you said, tell her (with appropriate pauses along the way) that:

- *The blood tests and the CT scan were done to look for an underlying cause* of her seizure.

'Some people inherit the tendency to developing fits, which usually starts very early in life. In others, it may be caused by an underlying medical condition. We did the blood tests and the brain scan to see if there was an underlying medical problem that caused your fits.'

- The blood test results are normal, but *the CT scan shows a possible growth*.

'Your blood test results are fine, but I am afraid the brain scan is not normal. [Momentary pause.] It shows an abnormality in the front part of your brain which the X-ray doctor thinks may be a growth.'

She says she did not expect this news. She asks what exactly you mean by *growth* and if it means that she has brain cancer.

Tell her that:

- *Not all growths are due to cancer.*

'I can see that you were not expecting this. A growth occurs when the cells in a certain part of the body start multiplying uncontrollably for no reason. It may or may not be due to cancer. Growths in the brain that cause fits are usually not due to cancer.'

- *The radiologist has suggested an MRI scan of the brain.*

'However, the scan that you just had, which we call a CT scan, is not good enough to tell us for sure if it is due to a growth. The X-ray doctor has therefore suggested another type of scan, called MRI, to get a better idea. You will be given an injection of a dye this time to improve the clarity of the pictures.'

Pause here for a while, and ask if she has any questions (*'Are you with me so far? Would you like me to go over anything once again?'*).

She says she is a bit worried but understands that all we know for now is that there is an abnormal area seen on the CT scan and the MRI will help clarify what it is.

Tell her that:

- *You will ask a neurologist to see her* after she has had the MRI scan.

'Once you have had the MRI scan, I'll ask our neurologist to see you. He will discuss the results of the scan and tell you what they can do about it.'

- *The neurologist is likely to recommend commencing an anti-epileptic drug.*

'The abnormality that we are seeing on the brain scan is possibly the reason for the fits, but the neurologist might suggest getting an electrical tracing of the brain to get a better idea of what is happening in the brain. The abnormal area in the brain could potentially fire again and cause fits in the future, so he may start you on a pill to reduce this risk.'

She asks if the growth can be removed.

- Tell her that *the neurosurgeon will discuss the treatment options with her.*

'We'll seek an opinion from our brain surgeon depending on what the MRI scan shows. He will discuss the treatment options with you. If the growth does not appear

like cancer and your fits respond well to the medication, he'll probably suggest repeating the scan at regular intervals to see if the growth is getting bigger. I don't think he will suggest an operation to remove the growth, unless it is getting bigger or you keep getting fits despite taking the medication. Most growths either do not grow at all or grow very slowly that they won't ever cause any further problems.'

- Ask if she drives a vehicle or has any hobbies that would pose a risk to her in case the seizures were to recur.

She says she drives a car. She does not have hobbies and does not do anything that would be considered dangerous.

- Tell her that *she must temporarily stop driving.*

    'You should stop driving for now. As I said, the fits could happen again. It could be dangerous if it happens while you are driving. You should also inform the Driving Vehicles Licensing Authority. You may be able to resume driving in the future once we know for sure that you won't get fits.'

She acknowledges your advice. She then tells you that she has had a headache for the last six months. She saw her GP about it a couple of times, but he attributed the headache to tension, as her workload increased about six months ago after a couple of her colleagues resigned. She wonders if the abnormal brain scan will explain her headache. She feels that her GP sat on the problem for too long and asks if an earlier brain scan would have prevented the fits.

- Find out more about the headache.

Ask if the headache is worse when she bends forward, coughs, or lies in bed (suggestive of raised intracranial pressure). Briefly ask if she has experienced any focal neurological features, like weakness or numbness in her limbs or face, visual loss, or change in speech.

She says the headache feels like a band-like sensation around her head. It is not worse on bending forward, coughing, or straining. Her sleep has never been disturbed because of the headache. She denies focal neurological symptoms. The headache comes and goes. It has neither worsened nor improved in the last three months.

Tell her that:

- *Her description suggests tension headache,* which is not related to the seizure.

    'Your description, indeed, suggests tension headache. I do not feel that it is related to the fits.'

- An *earlier scan was not indicated,* as there were no red flags prior to the occurrence of this seizure.

    'Your GP did not ask for a CT scan possibly because you did not have any worrying features. We don't scan everyone with a headache. A growth in the brain increases the pressure within the skull, which causes a headache that is worse with coughing or straining or when lying in bed. A growth can sometimes press on the structures in the brain

and make your limbs and face weak or numb. In some people, it can affect the vision or speech. You had none of these symptoms. However, please feel free to write to the manager at the clinic to hear your GP's point of view.'

End the consultation by summarising the main points. Reiterate to her that the CT scan findings are only suspicious and they have not confirmed the presence of a growth (*'Let's not jump to any conclusions until you have had the MRI scan, which we will try to get as soon as possible'*). Tell her that the neurologist will see her after she has had the MRI scan but she can ask to speak to you if she has further questions in the meantime.

SUMMARY

This scenario tests your skills in conveying an abnormal CT scan result and discussing the next steps. You will be expected to:

- Explain to her in layman's terms that the shaking of her limb was most likely due to a focal seizure.
- Tell her that the CT scan of the brain shows an abnormality, which may be a growth, and the radiologist has recommended an MRI scan to clarify this.

Do not make the mistake of saying that the CT scan shows cancer.

- Manage her emotions appropriately.
- Tell her what will happen next.

You will be asking a neurologist to see her. He might organise an electroencephalogram and commence her on anti-epileptic drug therapy.

- Tell her that the neurosurgeon will discuss the treatment options.
- Tell her that she must temporarily stop driving.
- Tell her that her description of the headache is in keeping with tension, so an earlier scan was not warranted.

The 22-Year-Old Woman with Type 1 Diabetes

This previously healthy 22-year-old engineering student was admitted to the acute medical unit yesterday (it was a Saturday) with a short history of abdominal pain, vomiting, and polyuria. At the time of admission, she was tachycardic, tachypnoeic, and hypotensive. Her abdomen was soft and non-tender. Physical examination was otherwise unremarkable.

Her blood tests showed severe hyperglycaemia, elevated serum β-hydroxybutyrate, and metabolic acidosis, in keeping with diabetic ketoacidosis (DKA). Her blood counts, liver function tests, serum creatinine, electrolytes, chest X-ray, 12-lead electrocardiogram, and urinalysis were all normal. Urine pregnancy test was negative.

She has remarkably improved in the last 24 hours with fluid resuscitation and fixed-dose insulin infusion. Her vital signs are now normal. Her blood glucose has normalised, and the ketonae-mia and metabolic acidosis have resolved. She has just been switched to subcutaneous insulin. Although the result of her glutamic acid decarboxylase (GAD) antibody test is still awaited, the impression of the team is that she has developed type 1 diabetes.

She feels that the medical team has got the diagnosis wrong. She has been referred to the diabetes specialist team, but they can only see her on Monday morning. The nurse asks if you could talk to her. You are the medical registrar on call.

When you walk into the room, you see a young woman of moderate build who is comfortable at rest.

- After introducing yourself, ask how she is and what she has been told so far. Find out why she feels that the team has got the diagnosis wrong.

She starts talking in an angry tone. She says the doctor who saw her the previous day told her that she has developed diabetes. She feels that it cannot be correct, as she thought diabetes was an old person's disease. She knows a few people with diabetes, and none of them are younger than 50. She wonders if they even knew that she was only 22! The other doctor spoke to her for about ten minutes, but she did not catch much of what he said.

It is not surprising that she did not catch much of what the other doctor told her. She was in the acute phase of her illness on the previous day and in an unfamiliar environment,

DOI: 10.1201/9781003533337-3

which would have made it difficult for her to process the information. There are several management issues to cover when you see someone with a new diagnosis of diabetes. However, as the diabetes specialist team is coming to see her the following morning, you should mainly use the time to (1) listen to her concerns sympathetically, (2) clear up her misconceptions, and (3) answer any questions that she asks about her diagnosis or treatment.

Type 1 diabetes (T1DM) results from failure of the β cells to produce insulin. About 90% of the cases of T1DM are caused by autoimmunity (type 1A), and the remaining 10% are idiopathic (type 1B). Patients with T1DM are usually young and thin, with no features of insulin resistance. DKA may be the first presentation. The presence of autoantibodies like GAD would point to T1DM, type 1A. The absence of antibodies would not rule out T1DM and may point to type 1B or type 2 diabetes (T2DM).

T2DM results from insulin resistance, which may eventually lead to insulin deficiency. It is by far the most common type of diabetes, accounting for about 90–95% of the cases. It usually begins insidiously, and there may be other features of hyperinsulinaemia, like central obesity, hypertension, dyslipidaemia, non-alcoholic fatty liver disease, or acanthosis nigricans. With the rising prevalence of obesity among young adults, it may be challenging to sometimes distinguish between T1 and T2DM. In this patient, the clinical presentation points more to T1DM, as (1) she is not overweight, (2) she has presented with diabetic ketoacidosis at onset, and (3) there are no overt features of insulin resistance.

- Acknowledge her frustration, and ask what she understands by diabetes.

  'I can see that you are upset. I'll try my best to explain what your problem is. First, tell me what you understand by diabetes.'

She says she knows that people with diabetes have a high blood sugar but not much beyond that. Her grandmother is a diabetic. She has seen her pricking the finger to check her blood sugar regularly.

Tell her (with appropriate pauses along the way to check her understanding) that:

- **Young people can also develop diabetes.**

  'Yes, correct. Diabetes means high blood sugar. We have an organ here in the upper part of the tummy called pancreas. The pancreas makes a hormone called insulin. Insulin helps our body use the sugars and produce energy.
  'Diabetes occurs either because the pancreas does not make any insulin or it makes some insulin but the insulin does not work properly. In the common type of diabetes that occurs in older people, the pancreas still makes some insulin but the insulin does not work properly. Young people like you can also develop diabetes, but that is usually because the pancreas has stopped producing insulin.'

- Based on her presentation with ketoacidosis, **you are certain that she has developed diabetes**.

  'Your blood sugar level was quite high yesterday, so we have no doubt that you have developed diabetes. When the pancreas stops making insulin, the cells don't get enough

glucose. The body then starts to use fat to produce energy. The breakdown of fat produces a chemical called ketone, which makes the blood very acidic. You felt so sick yesterday because your ketone level in the blood was high.

'When there is too much sugar in the blood, some of it leaks into the urine and pulls out extra water, which is why you were passing too much urine. You had lost a lot of fluids from your body because of this. The insulin that we are giving you has helped bring the blood sugar down, and I am glad to see that you are better now.'

Pause here for a while, and make sure she understood what you said. Invite any questions.

She asks why her pancreas has stopped making insulin.

- Tell her that her *diabetes is most likely due to autoimmunity*.

'Our immune system produces proteins called antibodies to attack our enemies, like bacteria and viruses. In the type of diabetes that occurs in young people, the immune system makes a mistake. It produces antibodies which destroy the cells in the pancreas that produce insulin. We do not know why the immune system makes this mistake in some people.'

She says the other doctor told her that she must continue injecting insulin for the rest of her life. She asks why she cannot take tablets like her grandmother.

- Explain why *she cannot take oral hypoglycaemic agents* (although you will be repeating yourself).

'The tablets generally work by either increasing the production of insulin or making the insulin work better. They won't work if the pancreas is not making any insulin at all. We suspect your diabetes is caused by lack of insulin, so the only option is to take insulin. Insulin cannot be taken by mouth because it is a protein and it'll be destroyed in the intestine.'

- Tell her that *you have requested GAD antibodies*, which will help confirm that she has T1DM.

'We have sent off a test to check for the presence of antibodies in your blood. As I just mentioned, these antibodies destroy the cells in the pancreas that make insulin. We find these antibodies in most people with the type of diabetes that results from lack of insulin. If the antibodies are present in your blood, it means that you can only be treated with insulin.'

- *Convey hope and optimism.*

'The diabetic nurse who is coming to see you tomorrow will teach you how to inject insulin. You may find this a little difficult to begin with – just like driving a car – but I am sure you'll get used to it very soon. I must also tell you that medicine is a rapidly advancing science. New treatments are being discovered all the time, so hopefully, you won't have to be on injections for the rest of your life. The rest of your life is a very long time in the field of medicine.'

She says she lives with her parents. She asks you not to tell them about her diagnosis. When asked for the reason, she says her mother will get very anxious if she learns that she has developed diabetes. She thinks she can manage this herself.

- **Encourage her to tell her parents.**

  'We, of course, won't, but I would strongly encourage you to tell them. Insulin can sometimes make the blood sugar level go too low. We call this hypoglycaemia, or hypo for short. It usually happens when you inject insulin and then don't eat on time or exercise strenuously. When the blood sugar level becomes low, you may feel hungry and start to sweat or tremble. When you experience these symptoms, you can increase the blood sugar level by consuming a sugary drink or eating something sweet. However, if the blood sugar drops to a very low level, you could become unconscious or get fits.

  'It is important for your parents to be aware so that they know what to do in case it happens at home. We can teach them to inject a medication called glucagon to increase the blood sugar level very quickly, as it has the opposite effect to that of insulin. It'll also make it much easier for you to manage your diabetes if you have their support rather than battling this all alone.'

She acknowledges your advice and promises to tell her parents at the right moment.

- **Ask about driving and recreational activities.**
  Note: You should tell her that you are asking about driving because she must temporarily stop driving and let the Driving Vehicles Licensing Authority (DVLA) know that she has started treatment with insulin (in the UK). It is important to know if she takes part in strenuous recreational activities because they may increase the risk of hypoglycaemia.

She says she does not drive. She tried to learn driving a couple of years ago but soon gave up because she was getting very nervous. She doesn't think she'll ever take up driving. She does not go to the gym or do anything that would be considered strenuous.

In the UK, car and motorbike drivers are given a group 1 licence, and those driving a bus, lorry, or taxi, a group 2 licence. Group 1 drivers must stop driving and inform the DVLA if they start long-term insulin treatment ($\geq$3 months), so that they can be given a restricted licence (a licence for 1, 2, or 3 years instead of one that extends up to the age of 70 years). The rules are stricter for group 2 drivers, who are given a licence for only one year at a time, provided that certain conditions are met.

Drivers on any form of treatment for diabetes must inform the DVLA if (1) they had even one episode of severe hypoglycaemia (requiring the assistance of another person) while at the wheel *or* (2) they had more than one episode of severe hypoglycaemia within a 12-month period at any time. Their licence will be revoked, but they can reapply after three months.

There are many countries where there is no legal requirement to inform the licencing authority. Regardless of the legal requirement, all patients on insulin who drive must be advised to follow the two-hour rule ('Check your blood sugar less than two hours before you start driving and every two hours thereafter if you are driving long distances'). They should be advised to drive only if the blood glucose is >5 mmol/L (take a snack before driving if it is between 4 and 5 mmol, and avoid driving if it is <4 mmol). They should keep some simple sugars, a glucometer, testing strips, and their personal identification in the vehicle at all times. They should be advised to pull up the vehicle to a safe location if they develop the warning symptoms and not drive for at least 45 minutes after correcting the hypoglycaemia.

- Stress upon her that *it is possible to prevent or greatly reduce the risk of long-term complications* with good control of her diabetes, but keep it brief.

  '*If you inject the insulin regularly and follow a healthy lifestyle, you can keep your blood sugar level under control. Diabetes can affect the kidneys, eyes, nerves, and blood vessels, but if the blood sugar level is kept under control, it should be possible to prevent or greatly reduce the chance of developing these problems.*'

End the conversation by telling her that the diabetes specialist team will discuss the treatments in detail and answer any other questions that she might have.

SUMMARY

This scenario tests your skills in talking to a young patient who is in denial after being diagnosed with a chronic disease. You will be expected to:

- Acknowledge her frustration and manage her emotions.
- Clearly explain in layman's terms that she has developed type I diabetes.
- Explain why she cannot take oral hypoglycaemic agents.
- Encourage her to tell her parents about her diagnosis and explain why.
Just telling her that you will keep the information confidential is not good enough.

- Provide the necessary advice if she drives a vehicle.
- Reassure her that long-term complications can be prevented or greatly reduced with good glycaemic control.

A similar approach should be followed when you talk to patients with a new diagnosis of other chronic diseases, like rheumatoid arthritis, systemic lupus erythematosus, multiple sclerosis, or inflammatory bowel disease. You will be expected to (1) discuss the test results and explain how the diagnosis was reached; (2) manage their emotions appropriately; (3) provide an overview of the treatments and focus on the positive aspects; (4) answer any questions about how the condition may affect their studies, career, family life, or recreational activities; and (5) tell them that you will refer to a specialist.

The 28-Year-Old Woman with a Positive HIV Test Result

This 28-year-old woman has recently accepted the position of an operating theatre nurse in your hospital. She previously worked as an operating theatre nurse in another hospital for over three years. As part of the pre-employment screening, she underwent various tests last week. Of these, her human immunodeficiency virus (HIV) test result has been reported to be positive. The result was negative when it was tested three years ago, prior to her previous employment.

She has been asked to come to the clinic to discuss the results of her tests. Your task is to break the news of the positive HIV test result and address her concerns.

- After introducing yourself, confirm her identity and make sure you are talking to the correct person.
- Start the conversation naturally. Ask about her job or why she decided to move. Then tell her why she has been asked to come to the clinic.

'As you know, we did some blood tests for you as part of your occupational health screening last week. I have the results of those tests. Can I discuss them with you now?'

- Tell her (after a warning shot) that *her HIV result is positive*.

'I'm afraid, your test results are not completely normal. [Pause momentarily before continuing.] Your HIV result has come back positive.'

It is best to break the news *before* obtaining any background information. You are seeing her after she has had the blood tests, so if you start the conversation by asking about high-risk sexual behaviour or needlestick injury, it will only make her more anxious, especially as she is a nurse with some background medical knowledge. It is also not appropriate to ask what she was expecting the results to show. When you give her a warning shot, it is better to say that 'the results are not completely normal' than to say, 'I have some bad news for you', as the treatments for HIV have vastly improved in the last two decades and they will no doubt continue to improve in the future.

- Do not continue talking after breaking this life-changing news. Allow her to digest this information. Watch her emotions. Say some comforting words.

'I am sorry. I know this comes as a huge shock for you.'

She becomes tearful. She says she got married only six months ago. She did not expect this news at all. She asks if you are sure that those are her test results.

- Tell her that it is indeed her result.

'Yes, I am afraid it is your result. I can see that you were not expecting this. A positive HIV result is life-changing, but it is certainly not the end of the world. Although there is no cure as yet, we have very effective treatments which can keep things under control.'

She wonders how she got this infection and straightaway starts to suspect her husband.

- *Check for risk factors for HIV.* Start with:

'Before I answer that, I hope you won't mind if I ask you some sensitive questions.'

Ask how long she has been with her husband. Is the intercourse protected or unprotected? Has she had other sexual partners? Has she ever injected drugs and shared needles? Has she had tattoos or body piercing? Does she recall sustaining a needlestick injury at her workplace?

She has known her husband for over three years, but they got married only six months ago. Her husband is her only sexual partner. The intercourse is unprotected, as they are trying for a baby. She had a boyfriend for over three years, but they split up more than five years ago. She has not had any other sexual partner. She has never used illicit drugs or had tattoos or body piercing.

She recalls pricking her finger with a needle in the operating theatre (OT) several months ago. There was some bleeding after the injury, but she washed her hands straightaway. She, however, failed to seek the advice of the occupational health physician, as it was a very busy day and she did not take it seriously.

Although it is not possible to conclude with certainty before obtaining a sexual history from the husband, the history of needlestick injury is relevant, as she did not seek immediate advice from the occupational health physician or take post-exposure prophylaxis. We can rule out her ex-boyfriend, as they split up more than five years ago and her HIV result was negative three years ago.

- Tell her that *she might have caught the infection from the needlestick injury.*

'It looks like you possibly caught the infection when you pricked your finger in the OT.'

She regrets ignoring the needlestick injury. She then asks you not to tell her husband about the positive HIV result, as she fears that he might leave her.

- *Encourage her to tell the husband* at the right moment.

'I fully understand. I know it's not easy. It is, however, important to test him for HIV, especially as the treatments for HIV are very effective in controlling the virus. If he is not tested, we'll miss the opportunity to treat him before it gets too late. I would strongly encourage you to disclose this to him. I am sure he will understand. Please don't blame yourself for this.'

Following your persuasion, she agrees to share this information with her husband. She asks if her lifespan is going to be shortened because of HIV.

- *Tell her that her lifespan will not be shortened* if the virus is kept under control with treatment.

  'Your chance of dying from old age is higher than that of dying of HIV. As I just mentioned, we now have very effective treatments to keep the virus under control. At the pace at which research in this field is progressing, I am sure the treatments will become even better in the future.'

She asks if HIV infection is the same as AIDS (acquired immunodeficiency syndrome). She says she knows that HIV can cause AIDS but is not sure at what point you start calling it AIDS.

- *Clarify the difference between HIV and AIDS.*

  'You are right. Not everyone with HIV has AIDS. The virus that causes HIV destroys a type of white blood cell called CD4 that protects us from certain infections. Once the CD4 numbers become too low, it'll increase your risk of getting some unusual infections that generally do not occur in people with a healthy immune system. We call them opportunistic infections. That's the stage when we call it AIDS, or acquired immunodeficiency syndrome. As the name implies, it is an acquired form of lowered immunity resulting from HIV infection.'

- Reassure her that *anti-retroviral treatments can greatly reduce the risk of progression to AIDS.*

  'The good news is that the treatments for HIV can greatly reduce the risk of developing AIDS. By reducing the amount of virus in the blood, these treatments will help stop the destruction of the CD4 cells and reduce the risk of getting opportunistic infections. I'll be asking for a few more blood tests to check the amount of virus in your blood and measure your CD4 count.'

She asks if she can continue to work in the operating theatre.

She is likely to perform exposure-prone procedures, which will increase the risk of exposure for patients under her care. In the UK, she can perform exposure-prone procedures as long as (1) she is on combination anti-retroviral therapy, (2) her viral load is undetectable, and (3) she is regularly monitored by an HIV specialist every three months. If her viral load increases at any point, she must stop working until her viral load is undetectable on two separate tests taken 12 weeks apart. The rules may be different in other countries.

- Tell her that it is best to *ask the HIV specialist about her employment.*

  'I'll be referring you to an HIV consultant. It is best to discuss this with them. As your work involves exposure to blood and blood products, there is a risk to the patients under your care if they are inadvertently exposed.
  'Once you start the treatment for HIV, you should get a blood test done to confirm that the viral load – the amount of virus in your blood – is below a certain level before you start working. You will be asked to get this blood test done every three months to

make sure the viral load is under control. If your viral load increases at any point, you must stop working straightaway and return to work only when the viral load returns to a satisfactory level. Alternatively, you can discuss with your manager and look for another suitable position. I am sure you can contribute well in another role too.'

She says she doesn't mind working in another location but will think about it and discuss with her manager. She asks if she can get pregnant and if her child is at risk of catching the infection from her.

- Tell her that *she can get pregnant and have children* but not until she has commenced treatment.

  'Yes, you can get pregnant and have children, but I would suggest that you put that plan on hold until you see the HIV specialist and start the medications. The medications are 100% effective in preventing the transmission of HIV to the baby. There is a very small risk of transmitting the virus to the baby through breast milk, so you should discuss with the HIV specialist if you wish to breast feed.'

- Her *husband must be tested for HIV*.

  'We should also test your husband for HIV. If his result is positive, he, too, will obviously need treatment. If his result is negative and your viral load is controlled with treatment, there is no risk of transmission to him. However, if he is worried about having unprotected intercourse with you, he can take medications to further reduce the risk of transmission.'

End the conversation by summarising the main points. Reassure her once more (*'I know this news has come as a huge shock to you, but I would like to emphasise that you can lead a normal life with some adjustments'*). Tell her that you will arrange the blood tests and refer her to the HIV clinic. If she has further questions, tell her that she can ask the HIV specialist, as it is not possible to cover all the issues in one consultation. Remind her to tell the husband so that he can get tested (*'Please let your husband know and ask him to get tested. I am sure you will feel a lot better once you have told him'*).

SUMMARY

This scenario tests your skills in communicating the diagnosis of a disease that carries a lot of stigma and has lifelong implications for her. You will be expected to:

- Gently break the news of the positive HIV result to her.
- Obtain background information about risk factors for HIV, and elicit the important history of needlestick injury.
- Encourage her to tell her husband so that he can get tested.
- Reassure her that anti-retroviral treatments are very effective in reducing the viral load and preventing progression to AIDS.

- Tell her that she can perform exposure-prone procedures provided certain conditions are met (in the UK).
- Tell her that she can get pregnant and have children. Once the viral load is brought under control, there is no risk of transmission of HIV to her sexual partners or future children.
- Tell her that you will arrange further blood tests to check her viral load and CD4 count, and refer her to an HIV clinic.

The 66-Year-Old Man with Advanced Pancreatic Cancer

This 66-year-old man was admitted to the acute medical unit (AMU) yesterday with a two-day history of yellowing of the skin and passing dark urine. He also reported upper abdominal discomfort, indigestion, loss of appetite, and unintentional weight loss of about 7 kg over the last three months. He denied any change in the colour of his stools, itching, or fever.

His background medical problems include diabetes mellitus, hypertension, and hyperlipidaemia. His regular medications are metformin, linagliptin, lisinopril, and atorvastatin. He drinks a couple of glasses of wine nearly every evening and smokes about five cigarettes a day. He used to work as a chartered accountant until he retired six years ago.

Examination at the time of admission revealed satisfactory vital parameters and scleral icterus. Abdominal examination was unremarkable, with no epigastric mass, hepatomegaly, or palpable gall bladder. His laboratory results showed serum bilirubin 80 µmol/L (normal <21 µmol/L), aspartate aminotransferase 72 U/L (normal 10–44 U/L), alanine aminotransferase 56 U/L (normal 10–34 U/L), alkaline phosphatase 612 U/L (normal 40–150 U/L), and serum albumin 41 g/L (normal 34–48 g/L). His CA 19-9 was 2,600 U/mL (normal <37 U/mL). Full blood count and renal function were normal. His glycosylated haemoglobin was 50 mmol/mol, indicating good glycaemic control. Chest X-ray was normal. His abdominal ultrasound scan showed dilated common bile duct; hence, an urgent pancreatic protocol abdominal computed tomography (CT) scan was requested.

The CT scan has just been reported as showing 'a locally advanced mass in the head of the pancreas encasing the superior mesenteric vein and blocking the bile duct, with multiple metastases to the liver and coeliac lymph nodes'. Your task is to discuss the results of the scan and the next steps with him and his wife. You are the medical registrar in the AMU.

- After introducing yourself, confirm his identity and the relationship of the wife. Tell him that you have come to discuss the results of his scan.
- Find out what he has been told so far. Ask if he has formed any ideas about what the scan might show.

He says he has had a discomfort and feeling of fullness in his tummy for the last three to four months. He has lost his appetite, and his weight has gone down by about 7 kg during this time.

DOI: 10.1201/9781003533337-5

He was ignoring these symptoms but decided to come to the hospital after his wife noticed that his eyes looked yellow.

The doctor who saw him yesterday told him that his liver tests were abnormal and arranged an ultrasound scan. This morning, they asked him to go for a CT scan. He wonders if the liver tests are abnormal because of his alcohol consumption, which he is happy to cut down. He is hoping to get better soon, as he and his wife have planned a grand trip for their 40th wedding anniversary later that year.

Although not confirmed histologically, his clinical presentation, CT scan findings, and the grossly elevated CA 19-9 are in keeping with advanced pancreatic cancer. You must use the time to tell him that (1) there is a very high likelihood of metastatic pancreatic cancer based on the scan and the blood test results, (2) further tests are required to confirm the diagnosis and assess the extent of spread, and (3) the gastroenterologist is likely to consider placing a biliary stent. The oncologist is best placed to discuss his treatment, but if he asks directly, you can tell him that a cure seems unlikely.

In real life, you must make sure your phone is silenced when you go to deliver bad news like this so that you are not interrupted until you finish. Gently break the news after a warning shot, convey the information exactly as described in the stem, speak slowly and clearly, provide the information in small chunks, and take care to avoid medical jargon. Do not give too much information all at once, as it is difficult for anyone in a highly emotional state to comprehend fully. Pause regularly to make sure he has understood what you have said. Respond appropriately to his emotions as you go along.

- After telling him that you are sorry to hear that he has been struggling, ask if he knows what the pancreas is and where it is located.

He says he knows that it is an organ that makes insulin. He is not sure where it is located.

Tell him that:
- The pancreas is located in the upper abdomen.

  'The pancreas is a fleshy organ that is located here in the upper part of the tummy. Apart from insulin, it also makes a juice that helps digest our food.'

- **His test results suggest a high likelihood of pancreatic cancer.**

  'I am sorry. The test results didn't turn out as well as we would have liked. [Momentary pause.] Your scan shows an abnormal growth in the pancreas. It is most likely due to cancer.'

They are both taken aback by this news. After quickly recovering, he asks how bad it is.

- Tell him that it appears that **the cancer has spread to the liver and coeliac lymph nodes.**

  'I am afraid the scan shows that the cancer has possibly spread to the liver and some lymph glands in the tummy.'

Do not continue talking after this, or just say, '*I can't imagine how difficult this must be for you both.*'

He asks if the cancer can be treated.

- Tell him that *further tests will be done* to confirm the diagnosis and assess the extent of spread.

'*We must first confirm the diagnosis of cancer before planning the treatment. We'll refer you to a bowel specialist, who may suggest getting a sample of cells from your liver or pancreas so that it can be looked at under a microscope. We call this a biopsy. It'll help confirm the diagnosis of cancer. We'll also ask for a scan of your chest and the lower part of the tummy to check if the cancer has spread to those areas. The cancer doctor will then plan your treatment based on the results of these tests.*'

He asks if an operation can be done to remove the cancer.

- Tell him that if the tests confirm that the cancer has metastasised, a *cure is not feasible*.

'*The specialist will discuss that with you. If the tests confirm that the cancer has spread outside the pancreas, I am afraid an operation to remove the cancer may not be an option.*'

- *The intent of treatment will be to prolong his life and control his symptoms.*

'*That does not mean that we can't or won't do anything. Apart from an operation, there are other ways to treat cancer. Although none of the treatments can get rid of the cancer, they will help you live longer and make you feel better.*'

He asks if this means he is going to die soon and how long you think he will live.

Tell him that:

- His *prognosis depends on the extent of spread and how well he responds to the treatments.*

'*It's difficult to predict. I am sorry for not giving you a straight answer. How long you will live depends on how much the cancer has spread and how well you respond to the treatments. The cancer doctor will be able to give you an idea once we complete the tests.*'

- The *team will also focus on improving his quality of life* regardless of how much time is left.

'*I must, however, tell you that we often get it wrong. We sometimes predict months and see people living for years. So rather than just worrying about how much time is left, we'll also focus on improving the quality of your remaining life and make sure you don't suffer.*'

He starts talking in a dejected tone. He asks if there is any point in getting more tests or seeing the specialists if they cannot get rid of his cancer.

Tell him that:

- The *oncologist will discuss the treatment options* for the cancer.

'I am sorry that you feel dejected. Let's take one step at a time. Let's do the tests first and see what they show. Even if we cannot get rid of the cancer, there is a lot that we can do to keep things under control and make you feel better. If the cancer cannot be removed, the cancer doctor will suggest medications to slow down the growth of the cancer and extend your life. We call this chemotherapy. The cancer doctor will explain this further.'

- The *gastroenterologist is likely to suggest placing a biliary stent* (draw a diagram to explain).

'The liver makes a green-coloured liquid called bile which flows along this passage into the intestine. The bile helps digest the fats in the food.

'Your scan shows that the growth is blocking this passage, which is causing the bile to leak into the blood. This is the reason you look yellow. In due course, the bile that leaks into the blood can make you itch. The blockage also increases the chance of infection in the passage. To reduce the risk of these complications, the bowel doctor is likely to suggest placing a tube called a stent to keep this passage open. The bile will flow freely into the intestine once this tube is placed.'

End the discussion by telling him that you would like to stop here, as you have given him a lot to take in. Tell him that you will arrange the scans and refer him to the gastroenterologist. The treatment will be planned by the oncologist once the diagnosis is confirmed histologically. Tell him that you would be happy to come back and talk to him if he has any further questions.

Although there are several more issues to discuss, it is best not to overwhelm him with too much information at this stage. Once the evaluation is complete, the oncologist is likely to discuss several other issues during subsequent consultations, including (1) chemotherapy, (2) the advantages of taking part in a clinical trial, (3) palliative measures, (4) advance care planning, (5) the need for pancreatic enzyme supplementation to improve his digestion, and (6) the chance of worsening diabetic control when the β cells of the islets of Langerhans are gradually destroyed by the cancer.

SUMMARY

This scenario tests your skills in breaking the bad news of advanced cancer. You will be expected to:

- Gently break the news after a warning shot, and tell him that the test results suggest a high likelihood of advanced pancreatic cancer.
- Tell him that you will arrange further tests to confirm the diagnosis and assess the extent of spread and seek specialist opinions.
- Tell him that if the tests prove that the cancer is advanced, the oncologist is likely to suggest chemotherapy to prolong his life. An operation to cure the cancer will not be an option.

- Tell him that it is difficult to predict how long he will live. The team will also be focusing on improving the quality of his remaining life.
- Tell him that the gastroenterologist is likely to suggest placing a biliary stent.
- Support the patient emotionally throughout the consultation.

The 74-Year-Old Man with Acute Myeloid Leukaemia

This 74-year-old man was booked for a coronary angiogram earlier this morning as he had been experiencing chest pain on exertion for the last six weeks. He also reported loss of appetite and loss of weight of about 3–4 kg over the same duration.

His background medical problems include diabetes and hyperlipidaemia. His regular medications are metformin, glipizide, and atorvastatin. He has been smoking about five cigarettes per day for more than 50 years but seldom drinks alcohol. He worked as a supervisor for a tyre factory until he was made redundant at the age of 56. He lives with his wife.

His physical examination this morning was unremarkable. His routine blood tests before the planned angiogram were reported as showing an elevated total white cell count of $75 \times 10^9/L$ (normal $4–11 \times 10^9/L$), haemoglobin 102 g/L (normal 130–170 g/L), and platelet count $164 \times 10^9/L$ (normal $150–400 \times 10^9/L$). The result was similar when the full blood count was repeated. His blood counts were normal when they were last checked just over a year ago. The peripheral blood film was reported as showing numerous blast cells with Auer rods, in keeping with acute myeloid leukaemia (AML). His liver function tests, serum creatinine, and coagulation screen were normal.

The cardiologist has therefore cancelled the angiogram and referred him to the acute medical unit for further evaluation of his leukaemia. Your task is to explain the diagnosis and the next steps to him.

- Introduce yourself, and check his identity. Start by asking what the cardiologist told him.

He tells you that he has been experiencing chest pain on exertion for the last six weeks. He consulted a private cardiologist, who recommended an angiogram because he suspected a problem with the blood flow to the heart muscle. However, he cancelled the angiogram this morning after seeing the blood test results. He told him there were some abnormal results on his blood tests which must be sorted first. He did not tell him anything else.

- Tell him that you have come to discuss the results of his blood tests. Ask about his loss of appetite and loss of weight, and if he has formed any ideas about those symptoms.

DOI: 10.1201/9781003533337-6

He says his appetite hasn't been good recently. Perhaps as a result, he has lost a few kilos over the last couple of months. He says his brother-in-law was diagnosed with cancer in his kidney about six months ago. He has been wondering if his symptoms, too, were due to some form of cancer. He asks what the blood tests show.

The detection of acute leukaemia on a routine blood test done for another reason is indeed unexpected. His angina was most likely triggered by the anaemia on a background of undiagnosed coronary artery disease. Although he has indicated that he was wondering if his symptoms were due to cancer, it does not necessarily make the task of breaking the bad news easier.

You should use the time to mainly let him know that (1) the blood test results show evidence of acute leukaemia, (2) he needs further evaluation for prognostication and planning the treatment, (3) you will refer him to a haematologist-oncologist, and (4) the oncologist is likely to recommend chemotherapy.

- After expressing your sadness for his brother-in-law, tell him that *his blood tests show marked leucocytosis and anaemia*.

  'In our blood, we have three types of cells: red blood cells, white blood cells, and platelets. Your blood tests show that you have too many white blood cells. Normally, there should be less than ten thousand white blood cells in a drop of blood, but your count is around seventy-five thousand. [Pause.] Your blood tests also show that you are anaemic. Anaemia means low haemoglobin level. Haemoglobin is the protein in the red blood cells that helps carry oxygen around the body.'

- His *elevated white cell count is caused by acute leukaemia.*

  'The white blood cell numbers commonly go up in people with infection but not to this level. Your results seem to suggest that there is a problem with the bone marrow, which is the soft inner part of our bones that produces blood cells.
  'The bone marrow normally produces immature blood cells called stem cells. The stem cells then develop into mature blood cells. Your bone marrow seems to have gone out of control. It is making an excessive number of stem cells which are not developing into mature blood cells. I am sorry to say that this is a form of blood cancer.'

Do not continue talking after this. Give him some time. Say something comforting (*'I am sorry to have given you this distressing news, and I wish things were different'*).

He remains calm and composed. He says he had a feeling that his symptoms might be due to cancer, so he is not completely surprised. He asks if it can be treated.

- Tell him that *you will be referring him to a haematologist-oncologist.*

  'We'll be referring you to a blood cancer specialist, who will arrange further tests to get more information about the cancer. The tests will help them plan your treatment.'

- *The oncologist is likely to recommend chemotherapy.*

  'The cancer doctor will probably recommend treating your cancer with medications. We call this chemotherapy.'

He says his brother-in-law received chemotherapy and felt very ill after that. He kept getting infections, so he decided to stop the treatment after some time. He asks if the side effects of the chemotherapy used for blood cancer are similar.

- Tell him that *the oncologist will take appropriate precautions to minimise his risk of infection.*

'There are different kinds of medications used to treat the various forms of cancer, and they are all broadly called chemotherapy. The medications used for blood cancer are different to those used for kidney cancer. Chemotherapy works by either killing the cancer cells or stopping them from multiplying.
  'They cause side effects because it's not possible for them to selectively target the cancer cells alone. They also target some good cells. The risk of infection is increased because they reduce the production of healthy white blood cells. The cancer doctor will give you some additional medications to minimise this risk. I am sorry to hear that your brother-in-law suffered some side effects, but that does not mean that you, too, will get them.'

He asks if he can choose not to be treated with chemotherapy. When asked for the reason, he says he has had a fulfilling life and he would like to go peacefully when the time comes. He does not wish to suffer the side effects of chemotherapy or pay frequent visits to the hospital during his last days.

Tell him that:

- It is best to *discuss with the oncologist and take an informed decision.*

'Might I suggest that you first discuss this with the cancer doctors? If, after listening to the pros and cons of chemotherapy, you prefer not to receive any treatment, they will, of course, respect your wishes. It is good to discuss with your family members, too, and see what they think.
  'If you choose not to receive any treatment for the cancer, I am afraid your lifespan will be significantly shortened. The cancer doctor will request further tests, which will help predict your response to treatment. Not all blood cancers are similar. How well you respond to the treatment depends on the type of blood cancer. If the results suggest that your cancer is likely to respond well to treatment, chemotherapy will help you live longer. So why don't you first get the tests done, see what the results show, and then take a decision after discussing with the cancer doctor and your family members?'

He says he will think about it. He then asks how much time you think he has got left.

- Tell him that *it is difficult to predict his prognosis,* as it depends on his response to treatment.

'It is difficult to predict accurately. It depends on whether or not you prefer to receive treatment for your cancer in the first place. I am guessing that an average person at your stage of illness who prefers not to receive any treatment will probably live a few months. It could be longer, if we are lucky. It could also be shorter. If the tests show that your cancer is likely to respond well to treatment, the cancer doctor is best placed to tell you how much your life can be extended.'

- The *team will also focus on his quality of life.*

  'Regardless of how much time is left, I am sure the cancer team will make sure you do not suffer. If you decide to not receive any treatment for your cancer, it does not mean that they'll stop caring for you. You will still receive the treatments to manage your symptoms and make you feel better.'

He asks if the chest pain that he was experiencing is related to the cancer.

- Tell him that his *anginal chest pain was probably triggered by anaemia* on a background of undiagnosed coronary artery disease.

  'I suspect you were getting chest pain because of a narrowing of the blood vessels supplying the heart muscle. Although the blood vessels may have been narrow for a long time, you probably started getting chest pain only recently because of the low haemoglobin. Haemoglobin, as I said earlier, is the protein that carries oxygen. I suspect your haemoglobin level is low because the cancer cells in the bone marrow are reducing the production of healthy red blood cells.
  'Whenever you exert, your heart muscle needs more oxygen. If the blood vessels are narrow and there is not enough haemoglobin, it makes it harder to supply the extra oxygen.'

End the discussion by summarising the main points. Encourage him to have a discussion with the oncologist and his family members before taking an informed decision regarding treatment. Tell him that the team will respect his wishes if he chooses not to receive any treatment for his cancer. Reassure him that regardless of his decision about treatment, the healthcare team will support him and ensure that he does not suffer.

SUMMARY

This scenario tests your skills in communicating an unexpected critical lab result. You will be expected to:

- Gently break the news that his blood test results show acute leukaemia.
- Outline the next steps, and tell him that you will be referring him to an oncologist, who will organise further tests for prognostication and planning the treatment.
- Give him a brief overview of chemotherapy, and address his concerns regarding side effects.
- Tell him that he has the right to decline any treatment for his cancer, but this must be an informed decision.
- Tell him that it is difficult to predict how much time he has left, and emphasise that the team will ensure he does not suffer.
- Explain that his anginal chest pain was most likely triggered by anaemia on a background of undiagnosed coronary artery disease.

The 27-Year-Old Woman with Possible Coeliac Disease

This 27-year-old woman was referred to the acute medical unit (AMU) two days ago as her blood tests showed severe microcytic hypochromic anaemia, with haemoglobin of 56 g/L.

She reported a three-month history of increasing tiredness and difficulty in performing household chores, prior to which she was in good health. She was also struggling to cope at work, which was office-based. She denied menorrhagia, bleeding from other sites, or gastrointestinal symptoms. Physical examination at the time of admission did not reveal any abnormal signs. Further investigations in the AMU showed low serum iron and low ferritin, in keeping with iron deficiency. Her white blood cell and platelet counts, peripheral blood film, vitamin B_{12} and folate, random glucose, thyroid-stimulating hormone, liver function tests, and serum creatinine were all normal.

She was given two units of blood transfusion yesterday, following which her haemoglobin has improved to 80 mg/L. Her IgA tissue transglutaminase (TTG) antibody has just been reported as positive (>10.0 U/mL). You are the medical registrar in the AMU. Your task is to discuss the test results and further management with her.

- Introduce yourself, and confirm her identity. Tell her that you have come to discuss the results of her blood tests.
- Ask what she has been told so far. Confirm that she has never had any symptoms apart from tiredness.

She says she is aware that her blood tests showed anaemia. The doctor who saw her at the time of admission told her that he would arrange further blood tests to find out why she was anaemic and recommended blood transfusion to improve her blood count. She denies menorrhagia, bleeding from other sites, and gastrointestinal symptoms, like abdominal bloating or cramping, indigestion, diarrhoea, steatorrhoea, or weight loss. She asks if the blood tests have revealed anything.

Tell her that:

- Her *haemoglobin has improved* after the blood transfusion.

  'I am sure the blood transfusion will make you feel better. Anaemia simply means low haemoglobin level in the blood. Haemoglobin is the protein in the blood cells that helps

DOI: 10.1201/9781003533337-7

carry oxygen around the body. The haemoglobin for someone of your age should be more than 120, but yours was only 56 when you came in. After the blood transfusion, it has picked up to 80 now. Although not back to normal, it is enough to improve your energy level and make you less tired.'

- Her *anaemia is due to iron deficiency*.

'You are anaemic because of lack of iron. Our body needs iron to make haemoglobin. Your blood tests show that your iron levels are very low.'

- Her blood tests suggest that *she may have coeliac disease*.

'Blood transfusion will only temporarily hold the haemoglobin level. Unless we find the reason for the low iron and treat it, the haemoglobin will drop again. We therefore did some additional tests to find out why your iron levels are low. The results suggest that you may have a condition called coeliac disease. Have you heard of coeliac disease?'

She says she has never heard of it. She asks if it is something serious.

Coeliac disease is a gluten-sensitive enteropathy that occurs in genetically predisposed individuals. Ingestion of gluten, which is present in wheat, barley, rye, and oats, triggers an autoimmune response that results in small bowel mucosal inflammation, villous atrophy, and malabsorption. It can present at any age for the first time. The usual symptoms are indigestion, abdominal cramping or bloating, diarrhoea, steatorrhoea, weight loss, failure to thrive or growth retardation (in children), and fatigue. Some patients may be asymptomatic ('silent coeliac disease') or only present with extra-intestinal features, such as anaemia (due to iron or folate malabsorption), osteomalacia or osteoporosis (due to calcium malabsorption), arthralgia, dermatitis herpetiformis, infertility, peripheral neuropathy, ataxia, and hyposplenism. It may be associated with other autoimmune diseases, such as thyroid disease or type 1 diabetes. There is a higher risk of enteropathy-associated T-cell lymphoma, non-Hodgkin's lymphoma, and small bowel adenocarcinoma, but they are all fortunately rare.

Serological tests such as IgA TTG and endomysial antibodies (EMA) are useful for screening. The sensitivity of anti-TTG is around 95%. IgA levels should always be co-checked, as IgA deficiency may cause falsely negative anti-TTG and EMA. Even if serology is positive, the diagnosis must be confirmed by small bowel biopsy, which is the gold standard. Treatment is lifelong strict exclusion of gluten.

- Tell her (with appropriate pauses along the way) that *coeliac disease is caused by eating gluten*, which triggers an autoimmune response that leads to small bowel inflammation.

'Coeliac disease is not serious in that it is not a life-threatening condition. Our immune system makes tiny protein missiles called antibodies to attack foreign invaders like bacteria or viruses. The antibodies are not supposed to attack our own cells. In people with coeliac disease, eating a protein called gluten triggers the immune system to wrongly attack the bowel lining. The bowel lining gets inflamed and damaged as a result, making

it difficult to absorb the nutrients from the food. Gluten is present in foods like bread, pizza, pasta, Indian flatbreads like chapati and naan, biscuits, and cakes.'

- **The suspicion of coeliac disease is based on her positive anti-TTG result.**

   'We found an antibody in your blood that is seen in people with coeliac disease. We suspect this antibody is attacking your bowel lining and reducing the absorption of iron from your food.'

- **The diagnosis of coeliac disease must be confirmed by small bowel biopsy.**

   'To confirm the diagnosis of coeliac disease, we must take a sample of cells from the lining of your small bowel and look at it under a microscope. We call this a biopsy. We'll refer you to a bowel specialist, who will pass a long thin tube called an endoscope via your throat into the small bowel to obtain the sample. This test will help look for evidence of inflammation or damage in the lining of the small bowel.'

She says she did not expect this news. She asks if it is really necessary for the sample to be taken from the small bowel. She would like to first discuss with her husband and sister before consenting to it.

Tell her that:

- **It is best to be absolutely certain** before committing to lifelong gluten-free diet.

   'The treatment for coeliac disease is lifelong exclusion of gluten from the diet, which is quite a major undertaking. It is therefore important to be 100% certain that you have coeliac disease before committing to that. The biopsy will help confirm that the antibody is indeed causing damage to the bowel lining. The presence of the antibody alone is not enough to make a diagnosis. In about 5 in 100 people who have the antibody, we don't find any evidence of coeliac disease.'

- **Endoscopy can help exclude other causes of iron-deficiency anaemia.**

   'The endoscope has a tiny camera at one end which will help the bowel doctor look at the inner lining of your food pipe, stomach, and small bowel and make sure there is no other reason for the anaemia. Inflammation or ulcers in the stomach, for example, can cause tiny amounts of bleeding, leading to anaemia. By doing this procedure, we can rule out those causes.'

She says she understands but will run this past her husband and sister before taking a decision. She asks if she must stop eating gluten straightaway.

- Tell her that *she must continue to consume gluten until the endoscopy is done.*

   'Sure, please do discuss with your family members. Please let me know if you want me to be there when you tell them, so that I can answer any questions they may have.
   'You should not stop eating gluten, however, until the sample is taken from your small bowel. If you stop eating gluten, your immune system will stop making the antibodies.

The bowel lining will no longer be attacked, so the inflammation will heal, and we will never know if you had coeliac disease.'

She asks if coeliac disease can be cured.

- Tell her that *consuming a gluten-free diet is the only way to keep the disease under control.*

'We'll talk about coeliac disease in detail once we confirm the diagnosis. If you exclude gluten from your diet, your immune system will stop making the harmful antibodies. The bowel lining will no longer be attacked, and the inflammation will heal. The bowel lining will return to normal. As long as you avoid gluten, you can lead a perfectly normal life.
    'If you start eating gluten again, the immune system will start attacking the bowel lining, and the inflammation will return. It may seem daunting at first, but you can continue to eat so many foods, and there are plenty of gluten-free options too. Once we confirm the diagnosis, we'll talk about it in detail. We'll also refer you to an expert dietician.'*

End the discussion by summarising the main points. Tell her that you will refer her to the gastroenterologist once she has made up her mind, as it is important to obtain histological confirmation before embarking on a gluten-free diet. Let her know that you will be happy to come back and talk to her if she has any further questions in the meantime.

SUMMARY

This scenario tests your skills in communicating the diagnosis of a life-changing condition that is yet to be confirmed on biopsy. You will be expected to:

- Tell her that her anaemia is caused by iron deficiency.
- Tell her that her anti-TTG is positive, which suggests a high likelihood of coeliac disease.
- Clearly explain the connection between eating gluten and the autoimmune response.
- Explain why a small bowel biopsy is essential to confirm a diagnosis of coeliac disease.
- Tell her that she must continue to consume gluten until the biopsy is taken.
- Reassure her that although the disease cannot be cured, it can be kept under control with lifelong strict gluten-free diet.
- Tell her that the gastroenterologist and dietician will explain the condition in detail once the diagnosis is confirmed on biopsy.

A variation of this scenario is talking to this patient after the diagnosis of coeliac disease is confirmed by biopsy, although in real life, those patients are usually counselled by the gastroenterologist and dietician. The discussion would then be mainly focused on what she can or cannot eat and how she can get around the restrictions in eating out, socialising, and going on holidays.

She might want to know if her child, sister, or parents should be screened, especially as the disease can be asymptomatic and there is a 1:10 chance of the disease occurring among first-degree relatives. She should be told that the recommendation is to offer serological testing every few years for all first-degree relatives or, if this is not preferred, to do genotyping for HLA-DQ2 and DQ8.

Two other important management issues in coeliac disease are the need to (1) perform a bone density scan because of the increased risk of osteoporosis and (2) offer pneumococcal vaccination because of the association with hyposplenism.

The 30-Year-Old Woman with Tuberculosis

This 30-year-old Asian woman was admitted to the medical ward four days ago with a three-week history of productive cough, low-grade fever, and night sweats. She denied haemoptysis, chest pain, and loss of weight or appetite. She was previously in good health. She migrated to the UK from India about seven years ago soon after she got married.

There were no abnormal signs on physical examination. Her blood tests showed normocytic normochromic anaemia, low serum iron, elevated ferritin, and elevated erythrocyte sedimentation rate. The rest of her blood counts, blood glucose, and liver and renal function were normal. Her chest X-ray showed right upper zone infiltration. Her respiratory virus panel was negative. She was placed in a single room because of the suspicion of tuberculosis and commenced on amoxicillin–clavulanic acid to cover for bacterial pneumonia.

Her sputum results have just been reported this morning as showing acid-fast bacilli on the smear and *Mycobacterium tuberculosis* on the polymerase chain reaction test. Sputum culture results for tuberculosis are awaited. You are the medical registrar on the floor. You have not met her before, as you have just come back from your leave today. Your task is to convey the test results and discuss the further course of action with her.

- Greet the patient, introduce yourself, and confirm her identity. Tell her that you have just come back from your leave and, therefore, did not manage to see her earlier.

Note: In real life, you must wear an N95 mask when you see someone with active tuberculosis, but this is not necessary in the exam setting when you talk to an actor.

- Ask how she is and what she has been told so far.

She says she has been coughing and not feeling well for more than three weeks. She has so far been told that she has been started on antibiotics because her chest X-ray showed an infection. She feels no different than how she was at the time of admission. Her temperature still goes up in the evening, and she sweats a lot at night.

DOI: 10.1201/9781003533337-8

- Ask if she knows why she has been placed in a single room.

'I am sorry to hear that. We can hopefully make you feel better soon. May I ask if you know why you have been placed in a single room?'

She says she was told that tuberculosis must be ruled out. She knows that it is an infection of the lung but is not sure why she has been placed in a single room.

- *Explain why she had to be kept isolated.*

'You are right. Tuberculosis commonly affects the lungs. It is different from most other lung infections, however, in that it can spread to the others when you cough, which is why we had to place you in a single room. Tuberculosis usually affects the upper part of the lung, and the cough lasts longer than a few weeks. We wanted to test you for tuberculosis because you had been coughing for more than three weeks and your chest X-ray showed an infection in the upper part of your right lung.'

Note: Say 'We had to place you in a single room', not 'We had to keep you isolated'.

- Then tell her that her **sputum result shows evidence of *Mycobacterium tuberculosis*.**

'The result of your phlegm test is back. [Pause.] I am afraid it shows that you do have tuberculosis.'

Among infectious diseases, tuberculosis is the second-leading cause of death (after COVID-19). All patients with suspected tuberculosis must be isolated in a single room. Airborne precautions must be taken (1) until the tests rule out tuberculosis or (2) for at least two weeks after the treatment has begun for patients with active tuberculosis.

Once a person is exposed to *Mycobacterium tuberculosis*, the possible outcome depends on the immune response.

- In a small number of people, the infection may be completely cleared.
- In most people (>90%), the immune response contains the infection, resulting in the formation of a granuloma (latent tuberculosis infection).

The bacilli remain dormant for several decades and often for the rest of the person's life. However, if immunity is lowered at any point, the person may develop reactivation tuberculosis. Risk factors for reactivation include human immunodeficiency virus (HIV) infection, immunosuppressive therapy (particularly glucocorticoids or anti-tumour necrosis factor), diabetes mellitus, chronic kidney disease, and malnutrition. Patients with latent tuberculosis infection do not experience any symptoms, and they are not infectious.

- In some people, the immune system neither clears nor contains the infection, thus leading to primary active tuberculosis.

Patients with pulmonary tuberculosis (primary active or reactivation) present with symptoms, and they may or may not be infectious. The usual symptoms are chronic productive cough, low-grade fever (particularly in the evening), night sweats, weight loss, loss of appetite, and fatigue.

She is a bit taken aback. She asks if it can be treated.

Tell her that:

- *Tuberculosis can be treated.*

  'Tuberculosis can indeed be treated with medications, but they must be taken every day for at least six months. You will be given four different medications to take for the first two months and then continued on two of those for the next four months.'

- It is *important to remain compliant with the treatment* to prevent drug resistance.

  'It is important to take the medications every day without fail even if you feel better. The bacteria will otherwise become stronger and stop responding to the medications. We call this resistance. Resistance is a major problem in some parts of the world. It occurs when people do not take the medications regularly as prescribed. Once the bacteria stop responding to the standard medications, we must use other medications, which may or may not be as effective, and the duration of treatment gets prolonged. We can prevent this problem if you take the medications regularly without fail.'

    'Your phlegm sample will be tested to see if the bacteria will respond well to the medications that we plan to start for you. The result of that test will take about six weeks. We can, however, start the treatment now and alter it later, depending on the result of that test.'

She promises to remain compliant. She asks if there are any side effects with these medications.

The important side effects to remember are (1) peripheral neuropathy with isoniazid, which can be prevented by co-administration of pyridoxine; (2) hepatotoxicity with isoniazid, rifampicin, and pyrazinamide; (3) orange discolouration of body fluids with rifampicin, which can stain contact lenses; (4) the enzyme-inducing property of rifampicin, which can reduce the efficacy of oral contraceptive pill; and (5) retrobulbar neuritis with ethambutol. Pyrazinamide may increase serum uric acid levels, but it is not relevant in this patient, as gout is rare in young women. If aminoglycosides are used, she must be warned about ototoxicity and nephrotoxicity. All four drugs (isoniazid, rifampicin, pyrazinamide, and ethambutol) are safe during pregnancy.

- Before you discuss the side effects, *ask if she takes the oral contraceptive pill (OCP) or uses contact lenses*.

She says she has been sexually inactive since getting separated from her husband about a year ago. She does not take the oral contraceptive pill. She does not wear contact lenses either.

- Tell her about the *side effects of anti-tuberculosis medications*.

  'As I said, we'll be giving you four different medications. One of those can cause inflammation of the nerves, but we can greatly reduce this risk by giving you a vitamin pill called pyridoxine. The second one can change your sweat, saliva, or urine to an orange colour. I asked about contact lenses because the change in the colour of the tears can stain them orange. This medication can also make the contraceptive pill less effective.

Three of those medications can potentially cause inflammation of the liver, so we'll be checking your liver tests on a regular basis. The fourth one can affect the nerve at the back of the eye, so we'll be sending you to the eye clinic for a check-up before you start taking the pills. I'll give you a leaflet that outlines all these side effects.'

She wonders how she got this infection, as she has not knowingly been exposed to anyone with tuberculosis.

- Tell her that she has most likely got reactivation tuberculosis.

'You probably caught the infection many years ago when you were living in India. In most people who catch tuberculosis, the immune system does not clear the bacteria from the body and only manages to contain them. The bacteria remain in their body for the rest of their lives without causing any problems.

'When the immune system suddenly becomes weak for some reason at a later stage in life, the bacteria will start multiplying and cause problems. It's not always possible to say why the immune system becomes weak and allows the bacteria to become active.'

- You would *recommend the HIV test.*

'I hope you won't mind if we do the HIV test for you. HIV infection is one of the possible causes for the tuberculosis bacteria to become active, as it weakens your immunity. It's a good idea to do the HIV test for anyone who has been diagnosed with tuberculosis, as it can be treated. I'll ask our nurse to talk to you about this test in detail.'

If she has no further questions:

- Explore her social situation. Ask who lives at home with her.

She says she lives with her two children, aged 4 and 6. She has left them with her mother-in-law before getting admitted to the hospital.

- Tell her that *she must remain isolated for two weeks.*

'It is better for the children to continue to stay with your mother-in-law for at least two weeks after you start the treatment. This is to prevent the infection from spreading to your children. After two weeks, you can have them back with you. I hope this arrangement will work.'

She says her mother-in-law would be delighted to have them with her. She asks if she would have already spread the infection to her children and if they, too, should be tested for tuberculosis.

- Tell her that *there is no need to test the children* in the absence of symptoms.

'It is possible that the children have already caught the infection from you, but as I mentioned earlier, the immune system will clear or contain the bacteria in a majority of people. If the children are well and active as usual, there is no need to test them.'

End the conversation by summarising the next steps. Tell her that you will arrange the eye check-up, get the nurse to counsel her on the HIV test, and refer her to the respiratory physician. The respiratory physician will follow her in the clinic to monitor her progress and response to treatment. She can be discharged home soon, but she must remain isolated for at least two weeks.

SUMMARY

This scenario tests your skills in communicating the diagnosis of a communicable disease that requires strict compliance with a long period of treatment and some isolation precautions. You will be expected to:

- Gently break the news that her sputum result is positive for *Mycobacterium tuberculosis*.
- Explain the rationale for isolation.
- Discuss the importance of compliance with treatment and the side effects of common anti-tuberculous drugs.

Remember to ask if she takes the oral contraceptive pill. You may get an unsatisfactory mark if you don't.

- Offer the HIV test and explain the reasons.
- Explore her social situation, and explain the need for her to be isolated for at least two weeks after beginning treatment.
- Reassure her that her children need not be tested in the absence of symptoms.
- Tell her about the follow-up arrangements.

Case 8

The 34-Year-Old Man with Hypertrophic Cardiomyopathy

This 34-year-old man was admitted to the acute medical unit (AMU) this morning after an episode of syncope. He was walking to the train station when he suddenly fell and hit his head on the ground. He did not experience any chest pain, breathlessness, palpitations, or dizziness before he fell. According to the passers-by, he was unconscious for a couple of minutes. He did not shake his limbs or bite his tongue. He was exhausted after the episode but not drowsy or confused.

His past medical history is unremarkable. He had never blacked out before. He is not taking any regular medication. He does not smoke or use recreational drugs and drinks alcohol only during weekends. He lives with his wife and two young sons.

His vital signs at the time of admission were satisfactory, with oxygen saturation of 97% on room air, pulse rate 68/minute, blood pressure 126/76 mmHg, respiratory rate 16/minute, and temperature 37°C. A mid-systolic murmur was heard over the precordium. A part from some bruising over his forehead, there were no other injuries.

His computed tomography scan of the brain, chest X-ray, and blood tests have all been normal. However, his 12-lead electrocardiogram (ECG) shows left ventricular hypertrophy with strain and deep 'dagger-like' Q waves. His echocardiogram has been reported as showing asymmetrical hypertrophy of the left ventricle and interventricular septum with left ventricular outflow obstruction, in keeping with hypertrophic obstructive cardiomyopathy (HOCM). Continuous ECG monitoring has not revealed any arrhythmia so far.

You are the medical registrar in the AMU. Your task is to discuss the test results and the next steps with him.

Hypertrophic cardiomyopathy is the most common genetic disease of the heart, with a prevalence of about 1 in 500. It is inherited in an autosomal dominant manner. It causes asymmetrical hypertrophy of the left ventricle and interventricular septum. The latter may cause left ventricular outflow obstruction. Most patients remain asymptomatic or develop only mild symptoms. Symptoms may be due to (1) left ventricular failure (e.g. shortness of breath, paroxysmal nocturnal dyspnoea, orthopnoea), (2) left ventricular outflow tract obstruction (e.g. syncope), (3) arrhythmia (e.g. palpitations, dizziness, syncope), or (4) left ventricular hypertrophy, causing oxygen supply–demand mismatch (e.g. angina).

DOI: 10.1201/9781003533337-9

Management of HOCM should focus on (1) relief of symptoms with medications such as β blockers, calcium channel blockers, diuretics, and the myosin inhibitor mavacamten or, rarely, surgical or alcohol septal ablation of the septum; (2) prevention of sudden cardiac death in high-risk patients by placing an implantable cardioverter-defibrillator (ICD); (3) genetic counselling to screen first-degree relatives; and (4) provision of advice regarding cessation of driving and avoidance of strenuous exercise.

- Introduce yourself, and confirm his identity. Tell him that you have come to discuss his test results. Ask how he is.

He says he feels well now but what happened that morning was quite scary. He has never experienced anything like this before. He is keen to find out why he fainted and what the tests have shown.

- Tell him that his *syncope was due to reduced cerebral perfusion*.

'I am glad to hear that you are feeling well. It appears that you fainted because your heart did not pump enough blood to your brain at that time.'

- Tell him that *the echocardiogram shows evidence of HOCM*.

'We did the tests to find out why you fainted. The brain scan, blood tests, and chest X-ray are all normal, but the heart scan shows a problem. [Pause.] It shows that your heart muscle is thickened. Before I tell you what that means, let me briefly explain the structure of the heart. [Draw a diagram to explain.] Our heart has four chambers, two at the top and two at the bottom. The bottom chamber on the right side pumps blood into the lungs, and the one on the left pumps to the rest of the body through this opening called the aortic valve. There is a muscle that separates the bottom two chambers. We call it septum.

'Your heart scan shows thickening of the septum and the muscle that surrounds the bottom left chamber. The thickening of the septum is narrowing the aortic opening, which is making it hard for the blood to be pumped out of the bottom left chamber. I suspect you fainted this morning because your heart was not able to pump enough blood past this blockage. We have a long name for this condition. It is called hypertrophic obstructive cardiomyopathy, or HOCM for short. [Write down on a piece of paper.] Hypertrophic *means thickening,* obstructive *because there is an obstruction to the free flow of blood through the aortic opening,* cardio *refers to the heart, and* myopathy *means problem in the muscle. So it is a heart muscle condition that leads to thickening and obstruction.'*

He says he is concerned to hear that there is a problem with the heart. He asks if it is life-threatening.

- Tell him that *HOCM is life-threatening in only a very small number of patients*.

'It could be life-threatening but only in a very small number of people. The heart muscle cells are not properly arranged in HOCM, so the electrical signal that passes through the

heart muscle can sometimes move in a very erratic manner and suddenly make the heart beat very fast and irregular. It is possible that your heartbeat briefly became irregular this morning when you fainted. In extreme cases, the heart can stop beating. We call this cardiac arrest.'

He asks if anything can be done to prevent the cardiac arrest or irregular heartbeat.

- Tell him that *a cardiologist is best placed to advise him regarding his risk of sudden cardiac arrest.*

'I'll refer you to a heart specialist, who will tell you if your risk of cardiac arrest is high. There is a device that can be implanted in the chest in people with a higher risk of cardiac arrest. If the heartbeat suddenly becomes fast and irregular, the device can detect it and deliver a small amount of electrical current to revert the heartbeat to normal. The heart doctor will explain this further.

'We are now monitoring your heart tracing to see if your heartbeat suddenly becomes irregular again. It is possible to continue to monitor your heart tracing even after you go home by strapping a device to your waist. It will help the heart doctor decide if the device needs to be implanted in your chest.'

He asks if he will keep fainting because of the blockage in the heart.

- Warn him that *the syncope may recur.*

'It is possible that you will faint again. The heart doctor will probably suggest a medication to improve the pumping of blood through the aortic opening and reduce the chance of fainting.'

- Ask about driving, his job, and exercise routine.

He says he drives a car. His job is desk-bound. The only exercise that he gets is walking to the train station in the morning and back home in the evening, which is about 15 minutes each way. He does not go to the gym or play any sport.

Tell him that:

- *He must stop driving.*

'You should temporarily stop driving, in case you faint while you are driving. After discussing with the heart doctor, you should inform the Driving Vehicles Licencing Authority.'

- *He should avoid strenuous exercise.*

'You can continue to walk to and from the train station, but please avoid strenuous activities, like going to the gym or playing a sport, as they will increase your risk of fainting.'

He acknowledges your advice. He asks why his heart muscle has become thicker.

- Tell him that *HOCM is a genetic condition* that is inherited in an autosomal dominant manner.

  'The condition is caused by a faulty gene. It means there is a spelling mistake in one of your genes. You must have inherited the faulty gene from one of your parents. It is also possible that you did not inherit it from either parent and the fault in the gene only started with you.'

- Ask about his family members. Particularly, ask about history of sudden death or cardiac problems among first-degree relatives.

He says his father died in a road traffic accident when he was only 10 years old, and his mother died from COVID a few years ago. They did not have any heart issues, as far as he is aware. His father's brother died suddenly at the age of 26 more than 30 years ago. He learnt from his mother that he was on a holiday in Cyprus at that time and collapsed while jogging. His father's sister and both her children are well. His mother had no siblings. All his grandparents died of old age or natural causes. His two sons are aged 4 and 6, and they are both well.

Tell him that:

- *Each of his sons has a 1:2 chance of inheriting the condition.*

  'Each of your two sons has a one in two chance of inheriting the condition from you. The heart doctor will recommend screening your sons by doing an electrical tracing of the heart and a heart scan. Your father's sister and both her children should also be screened. I suspect your uncle who died suddenly had this condition.'

- *Genetic testing is possible*, but it may or may not be possible to identify the mutation.

  'The heart doctor might arrange a blood test to see if the spelling mistake in your gene can be identified. It may or may not be possible, however. If it can be identified, we can then check for the presence of that same mistake in your sons.
  'If the mistake is not present, it means your child has not inherited the condition, and we can clear him. If the mistake is present, we should keep repeating the heart scan at regular intervals. The heart scan should be repeated every few years, because people with HOCM are born with a normal heart and the heart muscle gets thicker only later in life.'

End the conversation by summarising the main points. Tell him that you will refer him to the cardiologist, who will discuss the next steps. He should be able to go home soon. Finish on a positive note by telling him that the treatments for HOCM are likely to advance further in the coming years.

SUMMARY

This scenario tests your skills in communicating the diagnosis of a genetic condition and the long-term implications for him and his family. You will be expected to:

- Convey the test results and explain the diagnosis of HOCM in layman's terms.
- Reassure him that sudden death occurs in only a small number of patients with HOCM. If his risk is deemed to be high, the cardiologist will suggest an ICD.
- Advise him to stop driving.
- Advise him to avoid strenuous exercise, as it can trigger syncope and arrhythmia.
- Briefly talk about the mode of inheritance of HOCM and screening of his family members.

A variation of this case is talking to a pregnant woman whose antenatal scan shows adult polycystic kidney disease (APKD). You will be expected to (1) explain the diagnosis to her, (2) discuss the possible complications of APKD, (3) obtain a detailed family history and tell her that her current and future children have a one in two chance of inheriting the condition, (4) discuss how her family members will be screened, and (5) tell her that you will arrange a magnetic resonance angiogram of her brain after delivery if there is a family history of intracranial haemorrhage (it can be arranged after delivery, as there is no urgency).

Section II

Counselling on Disease Management

The 22-Year-Old Man with Recurrent Episodes of Fainting

This 22-year-old man was admitted to the acute medical unit (AMU) after an episode of syncope in the supermarket. This was his third episode of syncope in the last 12 months. The first episode occurred in a train station, and the second in a shopping mall. All three episodes were similar in that they were preceded by several minutes of light-headedness, nausea, and sweating. They only happened when he was upright. There was never any jerking of his limbs, tongue biting, up-rolling of the eyes, frothing at the mouth, or incontinence. He did not experience chest pain, palpitations, or breathlessness prior to the episodes. The syncope was not brought on by exertion or rising from a supine position. He recovered consciousness in less than a minute on every occasion. He was exhausted for several minutes after the episode but never drowsy or confused. He did not seek medical advice after the previous two episodes.

His medical history is otherwise blameless, and he is not taking any regular medication. He does not smoke, drink alcohol, or use illicit drugs. There is no family history of epilepsy or sudden cardiac death. He is single and sexually inactive. He is looking for a job, having recently graduated in hotel management.

His physical examination was entirely unremarkable. There was no postural drop in blood pressure, irregular pulse, cardiac murmur, or neurological deficits. The 12-lead electrocardiogram (ECG) and echocardiogram were normal. Continuous ECG monitoring did not reveal any arrhythmia. His haemoglobin was 135 g/L. His presentation was felt to be in keeping with vasovagal syncope.

You are the medical registrar in the AMU. Your task is to explain the diagnosis and management to him and his mother, who has come to take him home.

- Introduce yourself. After confirming his identity and the relationship of the mother, ask what they have been told so far. If you wish to obtain a history, keep it brief.

The mother says she is concerned because this is the third time he has fainted in the last year. The doctor who saw him at the time of admission only told them that he was going to arrange some tests. He didn't say anything else. She wants to know why he keeps fainting and what the tests have shown.

Causes of transient loss of consciousness include syncope (reduced blood flow to the brain) and seizures (excess electrical discharge of cerebral neurones). His overall presentation is not in keeping with seizure. Although seizure can be non-convulsive and tongue biting is not always a feature, it is usually followed by a prolonged post-ictal phase. On each occasion, he has instantly recovered consciousness upon assuming the supine position, which is not what happens in a seizure.

The three most common causes of syncope are (1) vasovagal, (2) cardiogenic, and (3) postural. Of these, postural hypotension can be ruled out, as he is not in the right age group (it is more common in the elderly), his symptoms did not occur soon after he rose from a supine position, and his lying and standing blood pressure measurements have been similar. Cardiogenic syncope usually occurs suddenly and will not be preceded by a prolonged prodromal phase. He does not report associated cardiac symptoms, like palpitations, chest pain, or breathlessness, and there is no family history of sudden cardiac death. There are no pointers on physical examination, and his 12-lead ECG, echocardiogram, and continuous ECG monitoring have not revealed any abnormalities.

Therefore, the most likely cause is vasovagal syncope. Vasovagal syncope is characterised by the 3Ps (postural, provoking factors, and prodromal phase). Although benign, it can recur. Most patients respond well to conservative measures. The patient and his mother should be reassured of the benign nature of vasovagal syncope and given appropriate advice regarding prevention and management.

Tell them that:

- *His presentation is in keeping with vasovagal syncope.*

  'There's no need to worry. It's not serious. We suspect he keeps fainting because one of his nerves, called vagus, is very sensitive. Our heart is supposed to beat about 60–100 times a minute. When the vagus nerve is stimulated, it slows the heartbeat and makes the blood vessels wider. This causes the blood pressure to fall, which reduces the blood flow to the brain at that time and makes him faint. As soon as he falls to the ground and lies flat, the effect of gravity is removed, and the blood flow to the brain increases, so consciousness is restored very quickly.

  'We call this vasovagal syncope – vaso refers to the blood vessel, vagal is the name of the nerve, and syncope is the medical term for fainting. It is only a symptom, not a medical condition or disease. In people who are sensitive, the vagus nerve may be triggered by things like unpleasant sights or smells, having a blood test, standing for a long time in a crowded place, hot weather, skipping a meal, not drinking enough fluids, and so on.'

She asks how you can be so sure that the fainting was caused by a sensitive nerve and not some underlying medical condition.

Tell her that:

- *His description of the episodes is not in keeping with seizure.*

  'There are, indeed, other causes for fainting. Fits, for example, can make a person faint. Fits occur because of too much electrical discharge from the brain. People with fits usually

shake their limbs, bite their tongue, and become confused for several minutes after the episode. They don't regain consciousness so quickly. We are confident that his description is not in keeping with fits.'

- **His examination findings and the test results do not point to cardiac syncope.**

'An irregular heartbeat or a heart problem that obstructs the flow of blood from the heart to the brain can make a person faint, but we did not find any evidence of those conditions when we examined him. Fainting due to a heart problem usually happens suddenly and without any warning. It will not build up so slowly with the sick feeling, dizziness, and sweating. The continuous tracing of his heart and the heart scan have not shown any evidence of a heart problem, which is good news.'

- **There was no postural drop in his blood pressure.**

'Another possible reason is a drop in the blood pressure upon rising from a lying position, but this will make the person faint soon after rising, not several minutes after being in an upright position. It usually occurs in older people. We measured his blood pressure in the lying and standing positions, and there was no difference in the readings.'

He asks if he will keep getting these fainting spells and what he can do to prevent them.

- **Tell him that he is likely to get further episodes of syncope.**

'Yes, you are at risk of getting further spells, but there are a few things you can do when you know that you are about to faint. The fainting will never occur suddenly. Before you faint, you will always experience some warning symptoms, like giddiness, sweating, and sickness, as you may have already figured out. You should not ignore those symptoms. If you do, the blood pressure will fall, and you will become unconscious. You will regain consciousness only after you fall to the ground and lie flat.

'Try to go to a safe place as soon as the symptoms begin so that you don't hurt yourself in case you fall. Lie down if you can, and raise your legs to increase the blood flow to your brain. If possible, drink a couple of glasses of water. In case you are not able to lie down, you can either squat or sit somewhere and cross your legs. You can also squeeze the muscles in your buttocks and calves. It'll help tighten the blood vessels and push more blood towards the heart – just like how the flow of water increases when you press a hosepipe. You should get up slowly only when you feel well.'

- **Outline some measures to reduce the risk of syncope.**

'To prevent the fainting spells, you should make sure you eat regularly and drink enough water, to keep yourself well hydrated. When we are upright, the blood vessels tighten up to move the blood in an upward direction. Not drinking enough fluids can reduce the blood volume and aggravate the problem. Some experts also recommend increasing salt intake. Most importantly, you should understand what your triggers are and just try to avoid them as much as possible.'

The mother asks if there are any medications to raise the blood pressure and prevent the fainting spells.

Medications are used for vasovagal syncope only if there is no response to the conservative measures outlined earlier. The two most commonly used medications are midodrine and fludrocortisone. Midodrine is an α-adrenergic agonist that causes vasoconstriction, while fludrocortisone is a mineralocorticoid that increases renal sodium absorption to expand the plasma volume. They have a modest effect and should only be used in patients without hypertension, heart failure, or renal disease.

- Tell her that *medications are considered only if there is no response to the first-line measures*.

'There are medications that increase the blood pressure by tightening the blood vessels or preventing the loss of salt in the urine, but we generally use them in people who don't respond to the measures that I just outlined. Medications only have a modest effect and may cause side effects, so we should try the general measures first. Most people get better with the general measures alone.'

He asks if he can drive. He says he is scared that he might faint while driving.

- Tell him that *he can drive, but he must take certain precautions*.

'You can drive. There is no restriction for people with vasovagal fainting to drive. The driving restriction only applies to people with fits or fainting that is caused by an untreated heart problem. Your fainting is not going to happen suddenly without warning. The symptoms will come on gradually, so you will always know if you are going to faint.

'If you get symptoms like giddiness, sweating, or sickness, lower the windows and make sure you pull up in a safe place. Get out of the car to get some fresh air. Follow the steps that I outlined to increase the blood flow to the brain. If you go on a long drive, have someone with you, if possible, and take a break at regular intervals. Avoid overheating of the car, and make sure you drink enough fluids.'

End the discussion by summarising the main points. Reassure him once more that although vasovagal syncope can be scary, it is a benign condition. There is no need for further tests or specialist referral, and he can be discharged home. He should be able to prevent or manage the fainting spells with the measures that you have outlined. Tell him that you will provide some written information or refer him to some useful websites.

SUMMARY

This scenario tests your skills in reassuring a patient about a benign yet potentially recurrent problem. You will be expected to:

- Explain to the patient in layman's terms that his recurrent fainting spells are due to vasovagal syncope.
- Reassure him that his fainting is not due to an underlying medical condition and further investigations are not necessary.

- Provide some advice on what he must do during the prodromal phase to prevent syncope.
- Outline some measures to reduce the risk of recurrence.
- Tell him that medications can be considered if there is no response to conservative measures.
- Provide clear advice regarding driving.

A variation of this scenario is talking to a young patient with syncope who has features of Wolff–Parkinson–White (WPW) syndrome on the ECG. You will be expected to (1) explain the condition in layman's terms; (2) discuss the potential complications of WPW syndrome; (3) tell him that you will refer him to a cardiologist; (4) give him a brief idea of the management options, including pharmacological treatment and catheter ablation (specialist knowledge is not expected); and (5) ask him to stop driving and inform the Driving Vehicles Licensing Authority.

The 24-Year-Old Pregnant Woman with Suspected Pulmonary Embolism

This 24-year-old woman, who is nine weeks pregnant, presented to the emergency department (ED) earlier this morning with a two-day history of breathlessness on exertion. She denied orthopnoea or paroxysmal nocturnal dyspnoea, chest pain, palpitations, syncope, cough, haemoptysis, or leg swelling. She did not go on a long journey recently.

Of note, she developed an unprovoked deep vein thrombosis (DVT) of her right leg eight months ago. She was diagnosed with antiphospholipid syndrome on the basis of persistently positive IgG anticardiolipin and IgG anti-β2 glycoprotein I antibodies. There were no clinical, laboratory, or serological features of systemic lupus erythematosus. She was advised to take long-term warfarin but stopped taking it about four months ago of her own accord. Her job is office-based. She has been a lifelong non-smoker and teetotaller. Her family history is unremarkable.

Her vital signs at the time of arrival showed an oxygen saturation of 96% on room air, heart rate 108/minute, respiratory rate 22/minute, blood pressure 124/78 mmHg, and temperature 37°C. There was no swelling of either calf. Her heart and lung sounds were normal. Her blood count, liver function tests, serum creatinine, urinalysis, coagulation screen, chest X-ray, and 12-lead electrocardiogram were normal. Urine pregnancy test was positive. The D-dimer test was not done because of its unreliability during pregnancy.

You are the medical registrar on call. Your task is to discuss the plan for further investigations and management with her. Her husband is present with her.

- Introduce yourself. Confirm her identity and the relationship of the husband. Ask how she is, and obtain a brief history.

She says that she has been getting breathless on exertion for the last two days. She therefore decided to come to the hospital and get checked. She only found out last week that she was pregnant, which came as a bit of a pleasant surprise for them, as it was unplanned.

- After congratulating them, ask what she was told about the diagnosis of DVT and why she decided to stop the warfarin.

DOI: 10.1201/9781003533337-12

She says she was told that she had a blood clot in her calf. The doctor who saw her at that time told her that she must take warfarin for the rest of her life because of some abnormal blood test results. She did not clearly understand the rationale for continuing the warfarin indefinitely. As she was feeling well, she decided to stop taking it after a few months.

Pulmonary embolism (PE) is the most likely diagnosis because of (1) the background history of antiphospholipid syndrome and (2) her pregnancy, which is a prothrombotic state. The other common causes of breathlessness, such as pneumonia, pulmonary oedema, anaemia, and renal impairment, can be ruled out because of the absence of supportive clinical findings or abnormal test results.

She is at risk of recurrent thrombosis (both arterial and venous) and increased pregnancy morbidity due to thrombosis of the placental blood vessels. She should be counselled about the need to continue anticoagulation treatment for life because of the risk of recurrent thrombotic events.

- Tell her that *her breathlessness is most likely due to pulmonary embolism.*

  '*I suspect you are feeling breathless because of a blood clot in your lung.*'

- *Explain why she was asked to take the anticoagulant indefinitely.*

  '*People commonly get blood clots when they don't move a lot, for example, after a long flight or car journey, or if they are hospitalised and confined to bed for more than a few days. There is usually something that provokes the formation of a blood clot.*
  '*However, in some people, blood clots form without there being any provoking factor. I understand that the blood clot in your leg was unprovoked. If the blood clot is unprovoked, we then look for an underlying medical condition that may have predisposed to it. In your case, the tests showed that your immune system was producing some proteins we call antibodies that were making your blood very sticky.*
  '*Warfarin is a blood-thinning medication that reduces the risk of blood clot by making the blood less sticky. You were asked to take warfarin indefinitely because your immune system will continue to make the antibodies forever. There is a risk, therefore, of developing further blood clots if you stop taking it.*'

She asks if there are any tests to confirm the blood clot in the lung.

In pregnant women with suspected PE, it may be prudent to start with a venous ultrasound scan of the legs even in the absence of clinical evidence of DVT. If the DVT scan is positive, it obviates the need to perform a computed tomography pulmonary angiogram (CTPA) or a ventilation-perfusion (Va/Q) scan. Both are associated with some radiation risk (slightly increased risk of breast cancer for the mother from CTPA and slightly increased risk of childhood cancer for the baby from a Va/Q scan).

The standard management of pregnant women with antiphospholipid syndrome (persistently positive antiphospholipid antibodies and previous thrombotic event) is therapeutic dose of low-molecular-weight heparin and low-dose aspirin to reduce the risk of thrombosis and fetal loss. Confirming the diagnosis of PE is therefore only of academic value in her case and will not change the management.

Tell her that:

- *Imaging tests can help confirm the presence of thrombosis.*

'Blood clots usually form in the leg and travel from there to the lungs. We can do a jelly scan of your legs to check for clots – we call it ultrasound scan. It's the same kind of scan that we do on the tummy in pregnant women to check for the growth of the baby. It's very safe, and there is no risk from exposure to X-rays. However, the jelly scan may or may not show the clot in the leg.

'If we do not find a clot in your leg, the next step is to do a scan of the lungs, to directly check for a clot in the lung – we call it CT scan. CT scans use X-rays, so in case we decide to do this, your tummy will be covered with a shield to protect the baby. However, getting a CT scan slightly increases your risk of developing breast cancer in the future. The risk, however, is very small.'

- *You would recommend anticoagulant treatment regardless of the scan findings.*

'The CT scan will tell us if your breathing problem is caused by a blood clot in the lung, but it will not change the treatment. Even if the scan is normal, we would still recommend treating you with the blood-thinning medication, as you are at higher risk of developing blood clots.

'The tests are essential only if we suspect a large blood clot, as the treatment is a bit different and may involve doing a procedure to remove the blood clot. People with a large blood clot in the lung are quite unwell, with a low oxygen level in the blood and low blood pressure, so I think it is unlikely in your case. We can do the jelly scan first, as it is quite safe, and see what that shows. If the jelly scan is normal, shall we stop there and not do any further tests? What do you think?'

She agrees with your plan and says she is happy to start taking warfarin again without getting a scan of her lungs.

Tell her (with appropriate pauses along the way) that:

- *Heparin is the anticoagulant drug of choice during pregnancy,* as warfarin is teratogenic.

'Warfarin should not be taken during pregnancy, as it can cause birth defects in the baby. During pregnancy, we use another type of blood-thinning medication, called heparin. It's only available in the form of an injection. You'll have to inject it yourself beneath the skin over your tummy twice daily until the end of your pregnancy. Our nurse will teach you how to do it.'

- *Heparin is associated with some side effects.*

'Heparin can cause a few side effects that you must be aware of. I'll write them down for you later. Just like any other blood-thinning medication, heparin can increase your tendency to bleed. When you receive heparin for several months, there is a small risk of thinning of the bones. We'll give you a vitamin D tablet to take every day to reduce this risk. Some women report hair fall, but the hair should grow back once you deliver the baby and stop the heparin.'

- *She will be switched to warfarin after delivery.*

'Heparin must be injected every day throughout pregnancy. Around the time of delivery, we'll switch you to a different form of heparin that is given through the vein. In case you need a procedure to deliver the baby, this form of heparin is easy to stop, and the effects will wear off straightaway, so the risk of bleeding is minimised. After you deliver the baby, we'll stop the heparin and start you on warfarin. It is safe to breastfeed when you take warfarin.'

- *Warfarin will reduce her risk of future thrombotic events.*

'I would recommend taking warfarin indefinitely, except when you become pregnant again. It'll reduce your risk of developing blood clots in the future. You probably know about the INR value, which tells us how thin the blood is. The dose of your warfarin will be adjusted to maintain the INR between 2 and 3.'

Pause and check her understanding. If she has no questions, tell her that:

- *You will refer her to a haematologist, who is likely to recommend low-dose aspirin* to reduce the risks to the fetus.

'We'll seek the opinion of a blood specialist. Because of your underlying medical condition, there is a risk of forming blood clots in the blood vessels that supply the baby. This can reduce the blood flow and affect the growth of the baby, cause premature delivery or, very rarely, death of the baby.
  'The blood specialist is likely to recommend a small dose of aspirin to reduce these risks. It can be taken along with heparin. Aspirin is also a blood-thinning medication, but it works differently. It comes in a tablet form and is taken once daily.'

End the conversation by summarising the main points that you agreed on. Tell her that you would like to admit her to the hospital, arrange the venous ultrasound scan to check for DVT, start her on low-molecular-weight heparin, and refer her to the obstetrician and haematologist. You will come back and talk to her once she has had the DVT scan.

SUMMARY

This scenario tests your skills in communicating the challenges of diagnosing and managing PE during pregnancy. You will be expected to:

- Tell her that her breathlessness is most likely due to PE.
- Discuss the imaging modalities that are available to confirm the diagnosis.
- Tell her that you would recommend treatment with low-molecular-weight heparin and aspirin regardless of what the scan shows because of the background history of antiphospholipid syndrome.
- Tell her that warfarin cannot be used during pregnancy as it is teratogenic.

- Warn her about the side effects of heparin.
- Emphasise the need to continue anticoagulation treatment indefinitely because of the risk of recurrence of thrombosis.

A variation of this scenario is talking to a pregnant woman with suspected PE but *without* a background diagnosis of antiphospholipid syndrome. Here, you will be expected to:

- Discuss the imaging options (DVT scan, followed by CTPA or Va/Q scan).
- Talk about the pros and cons of both imaging modalities.
- Counsel her on anticoagulation treatment.

The treatment of choice is heparin, which must be continued for the duration of the pregnancy and at least six weeks postnatally (there is an option to switch to warfarin after delivery). Those who develop PE towards the end of their pregnancy may have to continue anticoagulation beyond six weeks postnatally, as the treatment should be given for a minimum total duration of three months.

Case 11

The 37-Year-Old Woman with Functional Dyspepsia

This 37-year-old human resources officer presented to the outpatient clinic a couple of weeks ago with a one-year history of intermittent bloated feeling in her upper abdomen and early satiation. She denied abdominal pain, heartburn, dysphagia, vomiting, haematemesis, melena, loss of weight, diarrhoea, or constipation. There were no functional somatic symptoms, such as painful periods, widespread pain, tiredness, jaw pain, or chest pain. She denied being depressed.

Her past medical and family history are unremarkable. She does not smoke or drink alcohol. She seldom takes a non-steroidal anti-inflammatory drug, and the last time she took one was more than three years ago, for a toothache.

Your colleague who saw her two weeks ago recorded in his notes that her abdominal examination was normal. He felt that her presentation was in keeping with functional dyspepsia. He ordered a urea breath test (UBT) and arranged a follow-up appointment.

She has come to the clinic today for her follow-up appointment. Her UBT is negative. Your task is to explain the diagnosis and management of her symptoms.

- Introduce yourself, and confirm her identity. Briefly ask about her symptoms and what she was told by your colleague who saw her two weeks ago.

She says she has had this bloated feeling in the upper part of her tummy for over a year. She feels full before completing her meal. Her symptoms have neither worsened nor improved during this time. The doctor who saw her the last time told her that her symptoms were due to indigestion and arranged the breath test. She is keen to find out the cause of these symptoms and get some advice on how to get rid of this problem. She asks for the result of the breath test.

This patient is describing dyspepsia, which includes a constellation of symptoms, such as (1) pain or burning in the upper abdomen, (2) bloated feeling in the upper abdomen, and (3) early satiation (feeling full even before completing the meal). In a small number of patients, these symptoms may be caused by peptic ulcer, *Helicobacter pylori*, or stomach cancer. The rest will be diagnosed with functional dyspepsia (FD). FD is a poorly understood condition that occurs because of a problem with the two-way communication between the gastrointestinal tract and the brain.

FD is diagnosed in the absence of red flags, such as (1) older age (≥55 years), (2) loss of weight, (3) dysphagia, (4) vomiting, (5) gastrointestinal bleeding or iron-deficiency anaemia, (6) family history of cancer of the oesophagus or stomach cancer, and (7) epigastric mass. Patients with red flags must be referred to the specialist for further investigations.

Those in whom functional dyspepsia is suspected do not need further investigations or specialist referral, unless the symptoms are refractory to first-line treatments or the diagnosis is in doubt. Patient education is the key to successful management of FD. It is important to listen to the patient, show empathy, and not be dismissive when dealing with patients who present with 'medically unexplained symptoms' like FD.

- Tell her that **the UBT did not show any evidence of *Helicobacter pylori*.**

'*My colleague must have told you that he asked for the breath test to check for bacteria in the stomach that cause indigestion. The breath test was fine. It means your indigestion is not caused by bacteria. If we had found the bacteria in your stomach, we would have treated you with antibiotics.*'

She asks if you plan to do further tests. She says her friend's father, who complained of similar symptoms, has been referred to the hospital for a camera test. She asks if you are going to do that for her.

- Reassure her that *she has no red flags to warrant endoscopy*.

'*The camera test involves passing a long thin tube into the stomach. It has a camera at one end to look inside and take pictures. We call this endoscopy. It is mainly done in people over a certain age, or those with worrying symptoms, to check for cancer in the food pipe or stomach.*
   '*You do not have any worrying symptoms, like weight loss, problem with swallowing, constantly throwing up, or passing blood in the stools. We can confidently rule out cancer in someone your age in the absence of these worrying symptoms, so there is no need for you to get the camera test.*'

She gets a bit disappointed when you tell her that endoscopy is not necessary. She asks how you will know what is causing her symptoms without doing further tests.

Tell her that:

- *Her symptoms suggest FD.*

'*I hear you. But let me explain. When we eat, food passes through our gut. [Draw a diagram to illustrate.] The gut includes the food pipe, stomach, and bowel. The gut is connected to our brain by nerves, and they keep sending messages to each other through these nerves. These connections help the food move forward through the gut and get digested.*
   '*I suspect your indigestion is caused by a problem with the way these messages are being transmitted between the gut and the brain. The stomach is not moving the food to your bowel in time, hence making you feel bloated and full even before you finish your meal. We call this functional dyspepsia. Functional means it is not due to a medical condition, like cancer or ulcer. Dyspepsia is the medical term for indigestion. We don't*

exactly know why some people develop this problem. There are many things that we currently do not understand about functional dyspepsia. We'll hopefully learn more about it in the future.'

- **FD is a very common problem.**

'It is a very common problem. About one in ten people in the population suffers with indigestion. Among those with indigestion, roughly about eight in ten will be diagnosed with functional dyspepsia.'

- **Further evaluation or specialist referral is not necessary.**

'As I do not feel that your indigestion is caused by some serious disease or medical condition, there is no need to do further tests or see a specialist.'

Further investigations are only required in selected patients. These may include (1) full blood count in patients ≥55 years of age, (2) coeliac screen in those with overlap of irritable bowel symptoms, (3) upper gastrointestinal endoscopy in patients with red flags for oesophageal or stomach cancer, and (4) abdominal computed tomography scan in patients >60 years of age with weight loss (to exclude pancreatic cancer). In all other patients, the recommendation is to *test* for *Helicobacter pylori* and *treat* if positive.

Management of FD should focus on lifestyle changes, including regular aerobic exercise, stress management, and avoidance or restriction of diets that trigger or aggravate the symptoms. Acid-suppression therapy with a proton pump inhibitor or H2 receptor antagonist should be tried first, failing which prokinetic drugs like domperidone or low-dose tricyclic antidepressants (e.g. amitriptyline) may be added. Medications only have modest efficacy, so it is important to stress to the patient that her active involvement is more important than any of the passive treatments that are offered by the medical practitioner. Referral to a psychologist for cognitive behavioural therapy is an option for patients who do not respond well to first- and second-line measures.

She asks if there is any treatment that will restore proper communication between the gut and the brain to make the problem go away.

- Ask about foods that trigger her symptoms and stressors at home or at work.

She is unable to relate her symptoms to a particular food. Her job is quite stressful. Her two teenage children have been driving her crazy, and her husband is not very supportive.

Tell her that:

- **There is no cure for FD,** but several measures can help greatly reduce her symptoms.

'I'm afraid there is no cure, which means we cannot take the problem away completely. There are, however, several things that can help greatly reduce the symptoms.
'Certain foods like spicy foods, caffeinated drinks, and citrus fruits are known to trigger the symptoms of indigestion. It may be helpful to maintain a food diary to see what kind of foods trigger your symptoms, so that you can avoid or restrict them. I'd also

recommend reducing your portion size and eating more often. Try to avoid eating too late in the evening, so that these symptoms don't bother you at night.

'I am sorry to hear about your stresses. Stress can indeed play a part in aggravating the symptoms of indigestion. I may not have an easy solution to all your problems, but certain things like regular exercise, yoga, meditation, listening to good music, or reading a book will help manage your stress to a certain extent.'

- **You will prescribe a proton pump inhibitor,** but medications alone are not sufficient.

'I'll prescribe a pill to reduce the acid production in the stomach, but medicines alone are not sufficient to tackle this problem. The lifestyle changes are more important. There are also medicines that help improve the movements of the stomach or work on the nerves to make them less sensitive, but we'll consider them only if you don't respond to these first-line measures.'

- **Improvement is a slow process.** There is no quick-fix solution.

'Most people get better, but it'll take time. If you don't respond to any of these measures, I'll ask for an opinion from a specialist, but I hope that won't be necessary.'

End the conversation by summarising what you agreed on and the plan for moving forward. Tell her that you will prescribe acid-suppressing treatment but medications alone are not sufficient. Ask her to work on the lifestyle measures and dietary triggers. Tell her that you will arrange to follow her up and consider further measures only if her symptoms do not respond to the first-line measures. Provide some written information or refer her to useful websites.

SUMMARY

This scenario tests your skills in communicating the diagnosis of a medically unexplained problem. You will be expected to:

- Reassure her that her symptoms are not due to an underlying medical condition and further investigations are not necessary.
- Help the patient understand the concept of functional dyspepsia so that she can self-manage her condition.
- Outline the management of functional dyspepsia, including lifestyle changes, dietary modification, and acid-suppression therapy.
- Let her know that you will consider second-line treatments or specialist referral only if the first-line measures prove unhelpful.

The same approach should be followed for other medically unexplained or functional somatic symptoms, like chronic widespread pain, irritable bowel syndrome, or primary headache.

Case 12

The 46-Year-Old Man with Poorly Controlled Diabetes Mellitus

This 46-year-old man was diagnosed with type 2 diabetes mellitus about three months ago, when he went for a routine health screening. His lipid panel at that time showed elevated serum low-density lipoprotein and triglycerides. His blood counts, liver function tests, serum creatinine, and urinalysis were normal. He was commenced on metformin 500 mg BD and atorvastatin 20 mg ON.

His past medical history is otherwise unremarkable, except for a tibial fracture after a road traffic accident many years ago. He smokes about 20 cigarettes a day and drinks a couple of beers every day. He drives a taxi for a living. He lives with his wife and two teenage daughters.

He has now come for a routine follow-up appointment to the outpatient clinic. His blood test result from this morning shows glycosylated haemoglobin (HbA$_1$c) of 70 mmol/mol (8.6%). His blood pressure is 124/76 mmHg. He is overweight, with body mass index of 29 kg/m^2 and waist circumference of 102 cm.

You are the registrar in the clinic. Your task is to talk to him about his blood test result and suggest measures to improve his diabetic control.

- Introduce yourself, and confirm his identity. Explain the purpose of the consultation, which is to review the control of his diabetes.
- Start with an open-ended question, and ask how he has been. Check his understanding of diabetes.

He says he feels well. He has never had any symptoms from the diabetes. He knows that *diabetes* means high blood sugar but not much beyond that. He was asked to attend an education session with a nurse after his last appointment, but he missed that appointment because of his busy schedule. He takes his diabetes tablets twice daily, and the cholesterol tablet at night, without fail.

Patient education and empowerment are key to achieving optimal blood glucose control and preventing complications. You should use the time to make him understand that (1) his diabetes is caused by insulin resistance (the contribution of insulin deficiency may be omitted to keep it simple), (2) his diabetic control needs to be improved, (3) there is a higher risk of long-term complications if the diabetes is poorly controlled, (4) insulin

DOI: 10.1201/9781003533337-14

resistance is related to unhealthy lifestyle habits, and (5) healthy lifestyle measures are as important as medications to improve his diabetic control.

It is better to convey a few key take-home points that he is likely to remember than to overload him with too much information during this appointment. The education should ideally be provided over multiple sessions, complemented by pamphlets or online material.

- Tell him that *his diabetes is caused by insulin resistance*.

'Yes, you're right. Diabetes means high blood sugar. The carbohydrates that we consume are broken down into sugars in our body. We make a hormone called insulin to move the sugars from the blood into the cells.

'There are broadly two types of diabetes. In the type of diabetes that you have developed, the body does not respond well to insulin. Therefore, the sugars cannot be moved into the cells and the blood sugar level goes up. Being overweight, not being active, and eating unhealthy foods are the major reasons for the body not responding well to insulin. The medicine that you have been prescribed to manage your diabetes works by making the body respond better to insulin.'

After checking that he understood what you said:

- Tell him that *his diabetes is poorly controlled*.

'The blood test that you had this morning, which we call the "H test", tells us how well your blood sugar has been controlled over the last three months. I am afraid your "H test" shows that your diabetes is not well controlled. The reading should ideally be below 53, but yours is around 70, which is quite high. We must do something about it.'

He says he knows that the blood sugar should not be too high but is not entirely sure why.

- Tell him that *there is a higher risk of long-term complications if the diabetes is not well controlled*.

'If the blood sugar remains persistently high for a long period of time, it could damage the tiny blood vessels at the back of the eyes, kidneys, and nerves. Possible consequences of this are loss of eyesight, kidney failure, and loss of sensation in the hands and feet.

'Diabetes causes hardening of the blood vessels that supply the heart and the brain. This increases the risk of heart attack and stroke. The blood vessels that supply the legs, too, can become narrow and cause pain and sores or ulcers in the legs. With good control of diabetes, we can greatly reduce your risk of developing these complications.'

Pause for a while, and invite any questions. Find out about his lifestyle so that you can offer specific advice. Ask about his diet and exercise routine.

He gets defensive and says he can guess what you are going to suggest. He says it is not easy for him to adopt a healthy lifestyle. His work schedule is erratic. He leaves very early in the morning and works until late in the evening. He comes home for a few hours at midday to take a break. He manages to have his breakfast and lunch at home on most days but eats his dinner at some fast-food place nearly every day. He admits that he tends to snack whenever he is idle. He has no time for exercise. He asks you to just increase the dose of his diabetes pills, as he has not had any side effects from them.

His lifestyle is clearly unhealthy, but we must realise that it is not possible for everyone to go for a regular brisk walk and eat healthy, home-cooked food three times a day. Cab drivers, security personnel, and shift workers have an erratic work pattern, which makes it challenging for them to follow a healthy routine. It is important to acknowledge this and show empathy.

You should avoid providing generic advice with a long list of 'dos and don'ts', as they are readily available in any patient information booklet or website. You should instead provide advice that is specifically tailored to him. He is more likely to follow your advice if you work with him in partnership and give smaller goals that are achievable.

- *Acknowledge his difficulties.*

   'I'd suggest increasing the dose of metformin, the diabetes pill, as you've not had any side effects from them, but that alone is not enough to control your diabetes. We must also focus on diet and exercise. The aim is to help you lose weight so that the insulin can work better. I appreciate that your daily routine is not easy. It's not possible for any of us to radically change our lifestyle, but let's try to modify whatever we can. Even a few small steps will go a long way to improving your health.'

- *Provide some dietary advice.*

   'For a start, I would suggest cutting down the consumption of simple sugars, processed foods, and junk food as much as possible. You should go easy on things like fried foods, crisps, pastries, candies, biscuits, carbonated drinks, and fruit juices. It's good to include fresh fruits and vegetables in your diet and to try oats or brown bread for breakfast instead of cereals or white bread. When you snack, you can try some healthy options. Even better if you are able to move your working hours around and eat more often at home. I'll refer you to a dietician, who can advise further.'

He cuts you off and says he would rather enjoy his life and go when he is 60 than live a long boring life up to 100.

- Tell him that *the complications of diabetes could worsen the quality of his life.*

   'I don't mean to scare you, but the end may not be sudden. It may be preceded by many years of suffering and poor quality of life because of the complications of uncontrolled diabetes – for example, paralysis of the limbs because of stroke; breathing problems from heart disease; lack of blood flow to the legs, resulting in amputation; loss of eyesight; kidney failure; pain and numbness of the hands and feet; increased risk of infections; and frequent hospitalisations. Food is only one aspect of life. It's a matter of getting used to a new lifestyle and a healthy routine. You don't have to do all this at once. You can take it a step at a time.'

He says he will try to follow your advice but there is no way he can exercise. He has no time for it. He is pretty much in his cab all day.

- *Provide some guidance on exercise that is tailored to his daily routine.*

'I hear you, but it is important that you move as much as you can. Being sedentary will make it difficult to control your blood sugar or cholesterol and increase your risk of heart disease several fold. People who are active tend to live longer than those who are sedentary.

'Exercise doesn't have to happen in a gym. Why don't you go for a short walk in the morning before you leave for work? Even 20 minutes of walking will do you some good. Take a short walk whenever you are able to at other times. Try to park your car farther away from the eating place when you go for dinner and walk from there. You can also do some simple exercises, like lifting a pair of dumbbells or pushing down on your toes to squeeze your calf muscles, whenever you are idle. Every little bit will help.'

- *Advise him to stop smoking.*

'Another important thing is smoking. I would urge you to stop completely. People with diabetes or high cholesterol are at a much higher risk of getting a stroke or a heart attack if they smoke. Help is available if you wish to quit the habit. I can pass you a pamphlet, and we can discuss it next time.'

End the conversation by summarising the main points and agreeing on a way forward. Offer to make an appointment with the nurse educator, as she will advise him on a lot of practical issues that you did not manage to cover. Tell him that you will increase the dose of his metformin but that, if his diabetic control remains poor, you will consider adding other oral hypoglycaemic agents. Give him some goals to achieve before his next appointment (e.g. lose 3 kg, cut down the cigarettes, less junk food, walk for at least 20 minutes every day).

There are several other issues to discuss, such as (1) home monitoring of blood glucose (generally more useful for those who are receiving insulin or oral agents that can potentially cause hypoglycaemia); (2) warning signs of hypoglycaemia; (3) sick day rules; (4) foot, eye, and dental care; (5) control of other risk factors, such as blood pressure and hyperlipidaemia; and (6) influenza and pneumococcal vaccination. These issues can be addressed during subsequent appointments or by the nurse educator.

SUMMARY

This scenario tests your skills in negotiating a management plan with a patient who has a chronic disease and a challenging work schedule. You will be expected to:

- Tell him that his diabetes is caused by insulin resistance.
- Explain the connection between unhealthy lifestyle habits and insulin resistance.
- Give him a brief idea of the long-term complications of poorly controlled diabetes.
- Acknowledge his difficulties, and provide specific advice that is tailored to his lifestyle and daily routine.
- Demonstrate that you are partnering with the patient.

Case 13

The 78-Year-Old Woman with Hyponatraemia

This 78-year-old woman with a background history of mild osteoarthritis of the knees and early macular degeneration was admitted two days ago. She tripped and fell at home, two days before her presentation, hitting her head on the edge of a table.

Her vital signs were normal. Apart from some bruising over her scalp, physical examination was unremarkable. A computed tomography (CT) scan of her head showed a small subdural haematoma. The neurosurgeon, however, did not feel that operative intervention was necessary. He suggested an outpatient appointment in his clinic in a month and a follow-up CT scan just prior to that appointment. Her blood tests at the time of admission showed a serum sodium of 124 mmol/L (normal 135–145 mmol/L).

There is no history of recent diarrhoea or vomiting, and she is not known to have heart, liver, or kidney disease. She is not taking diuretics or antidepressants. She is clinically euvolaemic. There is no previous serum sodium value on her record. Her renal function, serum potassium, blood counts, thyroid function, serum cortisol, and chest X-ray are all normal. Her plasma osmolality is 245 mOsm/kg (low), and urine osmolality 368 mOsm/kg (high). Her hyponatraemia is therefore attributed to syndrome of inappropriate antidiuretic hormone (SIADH) secretion, most likely secondary to traumatic brain injury.

She has been struggling to follow the advice to restrict her fluid intake, and her serum sodium this morning was only slightly better at 126 mmol/L. The physiotherapist and occupational therapist have cleared her, but her discharge has been delayed because of the hyponatraemia. Her daughter has asked to speak to someone from the medical team, as she wants to know why her mother has been asked to restrict her fluid intake to less than 1 L per day. The nurse tells you that she is quite inquisitive. Your task is to explain the rationale for fluid restriction to her.

Antidiuretic hormone (ADH) is secreted in response to a contraction of the intravascular volume, which may be due to (1) loss of both sodium and water, as in hypovolaemia (e.g. diarrhoea, vomiting, diuretic therapy), *or* (2) retention of sodium and water from the activation of the renin-angiotensin-aldosterone axis, leading to increased interstitial volume and reduced effective intravascular volume, as in hypervolaemia (e.g. heart failure, liver cirrhosis, nephrotic syndrome).

DOI: 10.1201/9781003533337-15

In SIADH, as the name implies, there is inappropriate ADH secretion in the face of normal intravascular volume. The ADH causes increased reabsorption of free water from the renal tubules, and therefore reduced water excretion in the urine, leading to decreased serum osmolality and increased urine osmolality. A diagnosis of SIADH should be considered in patients with (1) plasma osmolality of <270 mOsm/kg and urine osmolality of >100 mOsm/kg, (2) euvolaemic fluid status, and (3) absence of evidence of hypothyroidism and glucocorticoid deficiency (as they both cause euvolaemic hyponatraemia).

The aim of fluid restriction is to give her less water than what she is losing every day (urine output plus insensible losses) so that there isn't much extra water for the ADH to reabsorb and maintain or aggravate the hyponatraemia. You should use the time to explain the basic concept of SIADH to the daughter and how fluid restriction will help. As the nurse has told you that she is inquisitive, you can expect a lot of questions from her!

- Introduce yourself, and confirm her relationship to the patient. Tell her why you have come to talk to her, and find out what she has been told so far.

She says they haven't been told much other than that she must not drink more than 1 L of fluid per day. She says she would appreciate if you could explain why. Her mother does not speak English.

After apologising for the lack of clear communication, tell her that:

- *Her mother's serum sodium is low.*

'Your mother's blood tests show that her salt level is low. It should normally be more than 135, but her level was only 124 when we checked it two days ago. It has now slightly gone up to 126. We do not know if her salt level dropped only recently or if it has been low for a long time, as we do not have any previous values to compare with.'

- *Her serum sodium is low because of free water retention.*

'A low salt level implies that there is disproportionately more water in the body. Let's say if we pour 100 mL of water into a mug and add 5 grams of salt to it, there'll be 5 grams of salt in 100 mL of water. If we then pour another 100 mL of water into the mug, now there'll be 5 grams of salt in 200 mL of water, or 2.5 grams in 100 mL. You can see how the salt level goes down without removing the salt but by simply increasing the amount of water. This is what happens in people with low salt level. They simply have too much water, which causes the salt level to fall.'

She asks why she has got too much water in her body.

Tell her that:

- *Her water retention is caused by SIADH.*

'We have a small gland below the brain. This gland makes a hormone called ADH. The ADH helps us maintain the right amount of water in the body. It's important for us to maintain the right amount of water at all times, neither too much nor too little. [Pause.] When we lose a lot of fluid, for example, after a bout of diarrhoea or vomiting, the water *content in the body goes down. We then make more ADH. The ADH makes us pass less water in the urine in an attempt to minimise the loss of fluid and restore the water content in the body. [Pause.]*

'*Your mother is making more ADH, although there is no need for her to do so, because she hasn't lost any fluid. Her gland has been tricked into thinking that it must make more ADH. It is making her pass less water in the urine and retain more in the body. The extra water that she is retaining is causing the low salt level.*'

- **The traumatic brain injury is the most likely cause of her SIADH.**

'*We suspect she is making more ADH because of the head injury. There is only a tiny collection of blood around the brain, which in itself is not serious, but any injury to the brain can stimulate the gland to make more ADH and lower the salt level. There are also some medical conditions and medications that can do this, but we haven't found any evidence of those in your mother.*'

She asks if there are any dangers in having too much water or a low salt level.

- Tell her that **an acute and significant drop in serum sodium may cause cerebral oedema**.

'*It's dangerous only when the salt level falls by a huge margin over a very short span of time. That only happens in a very small number of people. If the salt level falls suddenly, water can enter the brain cells and cause brain swelling. It can make the person sick, confused, drowsy, or unconscious. In a majority of people, it's not dangerous because the salt level only falls by a small margin or it falls gradually over a longer period of time. The brain will then do a few things to keep the water out of its cells.*'

After checking that she understood what you said:

- *Explain why her mother has been asked to restrict her fluid intake.*

'*To sum up what I have told you so far, her salt level is low. Her salt level is low because there is disproportionately more water. We are asking her to restrict her water intake so that we can bring the salt level up. The idea is to make her drink less than the amount that she's losing every day so that there isn't any extra water for the ADH to hold back in the body. If she drinks more than what she's losing, the ADH will retain the extra water and continue to keep the salt level low.*'

- Tell her that **fluids include anything that is liquid at room temperature**.

'*Fluids include not only water, tea, coffee, milk, and fruit juices, but also soup, ice cream, and yoghurt. Anything that is liquid at room temperature counts.*'

She says she understands, but her mother has been struggling to comply with the advice to restrict her fluid. She asks if you have any suggestions to make her comply. In response to your question on why she has been unable to comply, she says she is just used to drinking freely all her life and finds it very challenging to suddenly restrict her intake. Moreover, no one clearly explained why she must restrict her fluid intake, so there was no motivation for her to do so.

- After apologising once again, *give her some tips to comply with fluid restriction*.

'I understand. It's not easy. I can come with you when you explain to her. Hopefully, she'll comply if she knows why she must drink less. It'll help if she spreads out her fluid consumption throughout the day rather than drinking too much in one go. It's a good idea to drink between meals rather than with her meals. You can give her a smaller cup and ask her to sip instead of gulp. If her mouth feels dry, she can suck on small ice cubes or rinse her mouth with water without swallowing. If the low salt level is because of her head injury, it should resolve soon, and she won't have to do this for too long.'

She asks how long it will take for the problem to resolve.

- Tell her that *you are hoping that her sodium will return to the normal range soon*.

'Assuming that the ADH production is because of the recent head injury, the problem will hopefully be resolved soon. There is a small chance that she has had this problem for a long time, which means it is not entirely related to the head injury. The salt level may then not rise to the normal range, in which case, she should restrict her fluid intake indefinitely.'

She asks if there are any medications to remove the excess water and quickly bring the salt level to the normal range.

In patients with chronic hyponatraemia, the brain cells pump out various osmoles into the extra-cellular compartment ('cerebral adaptation'). These osmoles help retain water in the extra-cellular compartment and prevent cerebral oedema. If the hyponatraemia is rapidly corrected in such patients, the osmolality of the extra-cellular compartment will rise suddenly, resulting in more water being drawn from the brain cells ('osmotic demyelination syndrome').

Tell her that:

- *Fluid restriction alone should suffice in a vast majority of patients.*

'We sometimes use salt tablets or medicines that stop the ADH from working, but there is no need to try them when someone is responding well to fluid restriction and there are no symptoms because of the low salt level. Her salt level is not too bad, and it'll hopefully continue to rise, so let's persevere with fluid restriction alone.

'We must try to raise her salt level slowly. If her salt level is suddenly increased, it can pull water from the brain cells and cause them to shrink. It could prove life-threatening.'

End the conversation by summarising the main points. Tell her that you will check her serum sodium on a daily basis. If the sodium is moving in the right direction, you will be able to discharge her home in a couple of days, even if the serum sodium is not back to normal. You will give a memo to request her GP to check her blood tests in a week or so. Remind her that she must repeat her CT scan in a month to make sure the subdural haematoma is not increasing in size before seeing the neurosurgeon in his clinic.

SUMMARY

This scenario tests your skills in helping a family member clearly understand a challenging problem in order to improve compliance with treatment. You will be expected to:

- Explain to her that the hyponatraemia is caused by SIADH, most likely secondary to head injury.
- Clearly explain the rationale for fluid restriction.
- Acknowledge her difficulties in complying with fluid restriction, and give some practical tips to improve her compliance.
- Reassure her that hyponatraemia is not dangerous unless there is a sudden and significant drop.
- Outline the next steps and her prognosis.

A variation of this scenario is talking to a patient with heart failure who is struggling to comply with fluid and salt restriction. You should (1) explain the rationale for fluid and salt restriction, (2) talk about the risks of fluid overload, (3) acknowledge the challenges in complying, (4) provide some practical tips to improve compliance, and (5) discuss the role of medications.

The 26-Year-Old Woman Who Has Had an Anaphylactic Reaction

This 26-year-old woman, who was previously in good health, was admitted last night after an anaphylactic reaction at a friend's place. She developed a widespread rash, swelling of the lips, giddiness, and abdominal cramping within a few minutes of eating shrimp. She denied shortness of breath, wheezing, throat tightness, or change in her voice. She was not known to be allergic to any drug or food and had never had any problems with seafood before. She denied taking any medication or over-the-counter preparations recently. Her family history was unremarkable.

When she arrived at the emergency department, she was not in respiratory distress. There was no stridor. Her heart rate was 96/minute, blood pressure 84/52 mmHg, respiratory rate 20/minute, and oxygen saturation 96% on room air. There was a widespread urticarial skin rash and angio-oedema in her lips. Her heart sounds were normal, and lungs were clear. Her abdomen was soft and non-tender. She was seen by the otolaryngologist, who ruled out upper airway compromise.

She was given 0.5 mg of epinephrine intramuscularly, along with 200 mg of hydrocortisone and 25 mg of diphenhydramine intravenously. She was commenced on fluid resuscitation. Her vital parameters rapidly improved, and her blood pressure rose to 118/78 mmHg. Hourly vitals were ordered. Her blood counts were normal, with no evidence of eosinophilia.

She has been stable since admission. Her vital parameters this morning showed heart rate 72/minute, blood pressure 124/82 mmHg, respiratory rate 16/minute, and oxygen saturation 97% on room air. You are the medical registrar on the floor. Your task is to update her on what happened last night and outline the next steps. Her husband is present with her.

- Introduce yourself, and confirm their identity. Tell her that you have come to talk to her about what happened last night and the next steps. Start by asking how she is feeling and what she has been told so far.

She says she is feeling much better. She is only left with a faint rash over her chest and tummy. Her lips look normal again. She does not feel giddy, and her tummy pain has gone. The doctor who saw her last night told her that she thought she had an allergic reaction to the shrimp, but did not elaborate further. She asks if you could explain what exactly happened to her and if it was something serious.

DOI: 10.1201/9781003533337-16

Anaphylaxis is a potentially life-threatening acute hypersensitivity reaction. The usual triggers are (1) foods, like shellfish, peanuts, egg yolk, or cow's milk; (2) medications, like penicillin or non-steroidal anti-inflammatory drug; (3) bee or wasp sting; and (4) latex. The first exposure to the antigen results in the production of IgE antibodies, which attach themselves to mast cells and basophils. If re-exposed to the same antigen, the antigen combines with the IgE, causing mast cell degranulation and the release of mediators, like histamine, leukotrienes, and prostaglandins. The combined effect of these mediators causes broncho-constriction, vasodilatation, and increased vascular permeability. Some patients have a bi-phasic response, with symptoms recuring about 8–12 hours later (in the absence of ongoing treatment).

Shellfish allergy is common and may develop for the first time in adult life. People with an allergy to one type of shellfish must avoid all other types of shellfish (e.g. lobster, crab, mussels, oysters, scallops) and shellfish products altogether for life, as tropomyosin, the major shellfish allergen, is present in all of them. You should use the time to (1) explain to her what an anaphylactic reaction is, (2) outline the treatments that she has received, (3) guide her on what she must do if she gets another attack of anaphylaxis, and (4) talk about how she can prevent an allergic reaction in the future.

Tell her that:

- *She had an anaphylactic reaction.*

  '*I am glad to hear that you are feeling better. Let me first explain what* allergy *means. Our immune system is meant to defend us from foreign invaders, like harmful bacteria and viruses. In people with an allergy, the immune system mistakenly treats some harmless proteins as invaders and tries to fight them off. We then say that the person is allergic to the harmless protein that their immune system reacted to in this manner.*
  '*What you had last night was a severe allergic reaction. We call it anaphylaxis. It happens when the immune system reacts to the harmless proteins that are present in certain foods and medications. In your case, the immune system thought the shrimp protein was harmful and it had to be attacked.*
  '*The reaction causes the body to release some toxic chemicals. These chemicals make the blood vessels wider, causing the blood pressure to drop. Blood vessels become leaky, causing the skin rash, swelling of lips, and tummy pain. In some people, the airways become tight, causing problems with breathing. We don't fully understand why some people develop this kind of a reaction.*'

- *Her anaphylaxis was most likely triggered by the shrimp.*

  '*We suspect your reaction was triggered by the shrimp, as that was the last thing you ate just before you developed the rash. Foods like shrimp, oyster, crab, egg yolk, milk, and peanuts are all well known to cause this kind of a reaction. The reaction will reoccur if you eat the same food again.*'

She says she likes seafood but has seldom eaten shrimp. She asks what she must do if she develops the same reaction again.

- *Tell her about the treatments she received last night.*

'Before I answer that question, let me first tell you what treatments we gave you last night. Your blood pressure was very low when you arrived. We gave you an injection called epinephrine [write down on a piece of paper] to tighten the blood vessels and widen the airways. We gave you an anti-histamine medicine to block the action of a toxic chemical that is released during a severe allergic reaction – it's the same kind of allergy medicine that you get in shops without a prescription – and also a steroid medicine to reduce the inflammation. We also gave you a lot of fluids to raise your blood pressure.'

- *Tell her what she must do if she gets another attack of anaphylaxis.*

'We'll give you a supply of epinephrine, the medicine that helps open the airways and tighten the blood vessels. It comes in the form of a pen, so we call it EpiPen. As soon as you notice the symptoms of allergy, like skin rash, swelling of the face, breathing problem, or giddiness, you must inject the EpiPen into your thigh muscle right away. We'll teach you how to do it.

'People have died from anaphylaxis, so please don't take this lightly. An allergic reaction can happen at any time, so you must carry the pen with you at all times. You should inject it as soon as you notice the first symptom. Don't wait to see if your symptoms get better. If your symptoms do not improve within five to ten minutes, you should inject another pen – the injection comes in a pack of two. Even if you feel better after injecting it, you should still call an ambulance and come to the hospital as soon as possible. The EpiPen is only a first-aid measure. The reaction may happen again after several hours, so it is important that you are closely monitored in the hospital.'

She asks what she must do if the reaction occurs in a public place, as she won't be able to take off her clothes to inject into the thigh.

Tell her that:

- *She can inject through her clothes.*

'That's a good question. The EpiPen can be injected through the clothes. Don't waste your time trying to take your trousers off before injecting. Every second counts. The needle is designed to even go through jeans, but it is better to avoid seams, pockets, or very thick clothing, like a winter coat.'

- *You would recommend carrying an allergy alert card.*

'A severe allergic reaction can sometimes make you unconscious. It's therefore a good idea to carry an allergy card with you at all times, with details of your allergy, so that passers-by know what to do. Some people prefer to wear a wristband or a bracelet. I'll ask our pharmacist to help you with this.'

She asks if this means that she can never eat shrimp again.

Tell her that:

- *The reaction can occur with all forms of shellfish.*

'I'm afraid you must avoid all forms of shellfish, like crab, oyster, mussels, and lobster, not just shrimp. The protein that we suspect your body reacted to is present in other forms of shellfish too. This is very important because, as I said, anaphylaxis can be life-threatening.'

- *She should carefully check food labels.*

'You should always read food labels carefully to confirm that there are no shellfish components among the ingredients. You can eat in restaurants as long as you are sure that the dish that you ordered was not cooked in the same pot or pan as the seafood. I would discourage you from eating in seafood restaurants, however, as there is a high chance of cross-contamination.'

- *You will refer her to an allergy clinic.*

'I'll make an appointment for you in the allergy clinic to see a specialist. They'll do some tests to confirm that you are indeed allergic to shrimp. It may be a blood test or a skin test. For the skin test, they'll place various substances at different spots on your skin. You will develop a reaction in the skin if you are allergic to a particular substance. The allergy specialist will explain this to you.'

She asks if there is any cure for her allergy.

- Tell her that *most people will have the allergy for life.*

'I am afraid there is no cure, but things might change with medical advancements in the future, so let's be hopeful. We cannot make your immune system un-learn what it has learnt – it thinks shellfish proteins are harmful and they must be attacked. A very small number of people may outgrow their allergies, but for most people, the allergy will remain for life. There is no problem as long as you avoid the food that you are allergic to.
   'Allergy specialists sometimes try to give a miniscule amount of the substance that the person is allergic to and gradually increase the amount in small increments over a period of several months. It can reduce the severity of the reaction, but it is not a cure in that it will not take the problem away.'

End the conversation by summarising the main points. Tell her that the pharmacist will come and train her to self-inject the EpiPen and you would like her to continue taking the steroid and anti-histamine for another three days. Tell her you will give her written information on anaphylaxis and arrange an appointment in the allergy clinic. She should be able to go home later that day.

SUMMARY

This scenario tests your skills in communicating the long-term management of a life-changing acute medical condition. You will be expected to:

- Clearly explain anaphylaxis in layman's terms.
- Explain the treatments that she received last night.
- Tell her what she must do if she gets another attack of anaphylaxis.
- Talk about the precautions she must take to prevent an allergic reaction in the future.
- Tell her that you will refer her to an allergy specialist.

You will receive an unsatisfactory mark if you do not (1) advise her about EpiPen and stress upon her that its prompt use is life-saving or (2) ask her to avoid all forms of shellfish and shellfish products in the future. Those are the two most important points to convey to her.

The 48-Year-Old Man with Alcohol Use Disorder

This 48-year-old man was admitted two days ago with a three-month history of gradually increasing abdominal distension and leg swelling. He denied breathlessness, orthopnoea, reduced urine output, or frothy urine.

His medical history is largely unremarkable, except for a calcaneal fracture that he sustained after falling from a ladder a few years ago and a frozen shoulder. He does not smoke or use recreational drugs, but his alcohol intake has been far above the recommended limits for several years. He runs a family business and lives with his wife and two teenage children.

On examination, he had signs of ascites and chronic liver disease. His abdominal ultrasound showed a cirrhotic liver, splenomegaly, and moderate ascites. His laboratory tests revealed a low platelet count, macrocytosis, low serum albumin, and elevated liver enzymes. Screening tests for hepatitis B and C were negative. His blood glucose and lipid measurements were in the acceptable range. Serum ferritin, ceruloplasmin, and prothrombin time were normal. An upper gastrointestinal endoscopy revealed oesophageal varices.

He was commenced on propranolol, oral thiamine, and spironolactone. Although his CIWA (Clinical Institute Withdrawal Assessment of Alcohol Scale) score was not above the treatment threshold, he was 'front-loaded' with a tapering dose of lorazepam as prophylaxis against delirium tremens.

He has already been told about the diagnosis of alcoholic liver cirrhosis and its complications. The consultant feels that he could be considered for a liver transplantation provided he quits drinking and stays sober for at least six months. Your task is to talk to him about his drinking problem.

- Introduce yourself, and confirm his identity. Ask how he is and what he has been told already.

Do not start the conversation by telling him that you have come to talk about his drinking problem.

DOI: 10.1201/9781003533337-17

He says he was told that his belly is distended because of fluid collection and the fluid has collected there because of liver damage from alcohol.

- Tell him that *you would like to talk about his alcohol consumption*.

  'I'd like to talk to you about your drinking habit, if that's OK with you.'

- *Estimate the quantity and frequency of drinking and the duration of alcohol use.*
  (What does he drink, how much, how often, and for how long has he been drinking?)

Note: Be aware that alcoholics usually understate the amount they drink.

The scenario clearly states that your task is to address his drinking problem, so you should stick to that and not talk too much about the diagnosis of liver cirrhosis. You should use the time to (1) establish that he is 'addicted' to alcohol, (2) discuss the ill effects of continued excessive consumption, and (3) outline the help that is available if he is willing to quit the habit. Do not try to tell him all that you know about alcohol, as there is only so much you can say in ten minutes.

He says he mainly drinks beer, whisky, or rum. Although he started drinking at a very young age, his alcohol consumption has steadily increased only over the last ten years or so. He is unable to quantify the exact amount he drinks, as it varies, but it is usually around five or six standard drinks every day.

For a long time, he only used to drink with his friends in the evenings, but for the last few years, he has been drinking at lunchtime too, and even when he is alone, as he experiences cravings if he doesn't. He says he is aware that alcohol can affect his health, but he is unable to control the habit. He admits that it is affecting his business and the relationship with his family.

The definition of a standard drink varies among countries, but it is generally equal to 12 oz (341 mL) of beer, 5 oz (142 mL) of wine, or 1.5 oz (43 mL) of hard liquor (e.g. rum, gin, whisky, or vodka). The risk of all-cause morbidity and mortality increases with regular consumption of more than 14 standard drinks per week in men or more than 7 standard drinks per week in women.

However, addiction is not defined on the basis of the number of units or standard drinks consumed in a day or week. Not everyone who drinks excessively is addicted to it. We call it addiction only when the person has the *compulsion* to drink through intense *cravings* for alcohol and becomes unable to *control* the habit despite the negative *consequences* to health (the four Cs: compulsion, cravings, control, and consequences). Other features of addiction include tolerance (diminished effect with repeated use) and occurrence of withdrawal symptoms upon cessation. This man clearly exhibits features of addiction to alcohol (the preferred term is *alcohol use disorder*) and has developed organ damage as a result.

- *Ask if he is willing to quit the habit.*

  'Your drinking is clearly affecting your health. Would you like me to talk about how you can quit the habit? Are you ready for a change?'

He asks if there is any point in cutting down now, as the damage has already been done.

- Clarify that *you would recommend abstinence and not just moderation.*

'It's never too late to stop. I would recommend stopping completely, not just cutting down. If you continue to drink, I'm afraid the liver damage will progressively increase and your lifespan could be shortened. We are thinking of referring you to the liver unit to assess you for liver transplantation, but the transplant doctors won't consider that unless you stop drinking and remain sober for at least six months.

'Alcohol affects not only the liver but also several other organs in the body, like the stomach; the pancreas, which is the big fleshy organ over here in the upper part of the tummy; the brain; the heart; bones; and nerves. It also increases your risk of developing certain cancers, high blood pressure, and mental health problems. You can considerably cut down the risk of developing these problems if you stop drinking.'

He says he appreciates your concern and understands that alcohol is bad for his health, but he really suffered during the pandemic lockdown when he was forced to cut down. He was getting shaky. He was anxious and irritable all the time. He experienced a fullness in his head. He wasn't able to sleep well. He is worried that all these symptoms will be much worse if he quits the habit. He doesn't think he can quit the habit after so many years of heavy drinking.

- Tell him that *you will refer him to an addiction treatment centre.*

'I hear you. I am certainly not suggesting that you should do this on your own. It's advisable to do it under medical supervision because you are likely to experience very unpleasant or dangerous symptoms if you suddenly stop drinking. I'll refer you to an addiction treatment centre.'

He asks what they'll do at the addiction centre.

There are three stages in the management of alcohol use disorder, including (1) treatment of the withdrawal symptoms, also known as detoxification treatment; (2) treatment of the addiction; and (3) prevention of relapse. The treatments can be completed in an inpatient or outpatient setting, depending on the patient type, amount of alcohol consumed, anticipated severity of withdrawal symptoms, comorbidities, and social circumstances.

Alcohol withdrawal symptoms should not be taken lightly, as they can potentially be life-threatening. The symptoms usually begin within 6–24 hours after the last drink, peak at 36–72 hours, and last about five to seven days. Features may include anxiety, restlessness, insomnia, tremors, sweating, nausea, rapid heart rate, high blood pressure, and in extreme cases, delirium, seizures, and hallucinations ('delirium tremens'). They are managed with a tapering dose of oral or parenteral benzodiazepine, like diazepam or lorazepam, as they mimic the effect of alcohol on the brain.

Once the patient is past the unpleasant withdrawal phase, the focus then shifts to the management of the addiction with a biopsychosocial approach. Biological treatments include drugs like naltrexone and acamprosate to reduce the cravings and maintain sobriety, while psychological treatments include cognitive behavioural therapy and motivational interviewing. The underlying reasons for the addiction are addressed, and the person is encouraged to join a mutual support group, like Alcoholics Anonymous (AA), to reduce the risk of relapse and maintain long-term abstinence.

Briefly tell him what to expect at the addiction treatment centre. Tell him that:

- *He will first receive alcohol detox treatment.*

   'The first step is to manage the withdrawal symptoms that you are likely to get when you stop drinking. Alcohol has a depressing effect on the brain. When you drink excessively, the brain produces some stimulant chemicals to balance the depressing effect of alcohol. If you suddenly stop drinking, the stimulant chemicals will take an upper hand and make you experience some troublesome symptoms, like shaking, sweating, and sickness. Your heart can start racing, and your blood pressure can shoot up. Some people are also at risk of getting fits or becoming confused and agitated. They may start to see things that are not there or feel bugs crawling on their skin – we call this hallucination.
   'At the treatment centre, they'll make sure you get appropriate medicines to prevent these symptoms – we call it detox. You'll need the detox treatment for about a week, until the brain realises that there is no alcohol in your body and it doesn't need to produce the stimulant chemicals anymore.'

- *Once detox is completed, he will go through a phase of rehabilitation.*

   'Once the alcohol is out of your body and they've managed the withdrawal symptoms, they'll move to the next phase, which is the treatment for the addiction itself. This phase will involve the use of medicines and counselling.
   'Your physical cravings will subside within a couple of weeks, but the mental cravings can last several months. The medicines will reduce these cravings and help you stay sober. Counselling will aim to change your thoughts, emotions, and behaviours that led to the drinking habit and motivate you to change. The treatments are very effective, but it'll take time. Countless people have been able to successfully quit the habit after going through programs like this.'

- *It is important to maintain abstinence and prevent a relapse.*

   'We must ensure that you not only stop drinking but also stay stopped. During counselling, they'll try to understand the reasons behind your addiction, which is important to stop you from drinking again. They'll teach you how to avoid tempting situations or what you should do if you face one. It's not easy to do all this on your own, so your family members will be invited to get involved, if you do not have any objections. You'll also be encouraged to join a support group. You must have heard of AA, or Alcoholics Anonymous – it's a voluntary organisation that includes members who have successfully quit the habit. You can learn a lot from the experience of others. You can help the others too.'

End the conversation by summarising the main points. Tell him that you will refer him to an addiction treatment centre once he has made up his mind. Emphasise that although it takes time, the treatments work. If he successfully quits the habit, it will have positive effects not only on his physical and mental health but also on his social relationships. Tell him that if he stays sober for at least six months, you'll refer him to a liver transplant unit. If he manages to get a transplant, he can start his life all over again.

SUMMARY

This scenario test$ your skills in communicating the ill effects of a long-standing addiction problem and its management. You will be expected to:

- Establish that he is addicted to alcohol.
- Explain the ill effects of alcohol, and assess his motivation to stop drinking.
- Provide an overview of the services that are available to help him quit the habit.
- Address his concerns appropriately, and show compassion.
- Demonstrate your knowledge of the alcohol detox treatment and the process of rehabilitation to treat the addiction and maintain long-term abstinence.
- Warn him about the dangers of trying to quit the habit himself without medical supervision.

The 28-Year-Old Woman with Possible Lupus Nephritis

This 28-year-old woman presented to the acute medical unit (AMU) this morning with a one-week history of leg swelling, facial puffiness, oliguria, and dark urine.

She was diagnosed with systemic lupus erythematosus (SLE) about six months ago. She had then presented with joint pains, photosensitive skin rashes and tiredness, with no evidence of internal organ involvement. The results of her lab tests at that time showed lymphopenia, anti-nuclear antibody 1/640, elevated double-stranded deoxyribonucleic acid antibody, and low serum complements. Antibodies to extractable nuclear antigens and antiphospholipid antibodies were negative. Screening tests for hepatitis B and C were negative. Her blood glucose, lipid profile, and vitamin D were normal. She declined low-dose prednisolone and only took a prescription for hydroxychloroquine. She subsequently did not attend her follow-up appointment to see the rheumatologist three months later.

Her medical history is otherwise unremarkable. She does not smoke or drink alcohol. She is single and not sexually active. She is the manager of a swimming club.

Her blood pressure at the time of admission was 150/100 mmHg. She had bilateral pitting pedal oedema up to the level of her shins. Her heart sounds were normal, and lungs were clear. Abdomen was soft and non-tender. The rest of her examination was unremarkable.

Her test results have just come back, and they show haematuria with red cell casts, dysmorphic red cells >20%, estimated proteinuria of 1.5 g/day, serum creatinine 176 µmol/L (previously normal six months ago), and serum albumin 28 g/L (normal 35–45 g/L). Her blood counts, liver function tests, and chest X-ray are normal. The ultrasound scan has been reported as showing normal-sized kidneys, with no evidence of obstruction. Urine pregnancy test is negative.

You are the medical registrar in the AMU. Your task is to discuss the test results, the most likely diagnosis, and the next steps with her.

- Introduce yourself and confirm her identity. Obtain a brief history, and find out what she knows about her condition.

DOI: 10.1201/9781003533337-18

She says the rheumatologist told her that had SLE. Based on what she told her, she knows that her immune system is attacking her own body. The rheumatologist suggested steroids, but she was not keen to take them because she was worried that she'll put on weight. She was given another pill to treat the SLE, but she did not take it. There is no specific reason for not taking it; she just didn't like taking medicines and wanted to see if the problem will go away on its own. She has never tried alternative treatments. She did not attend her follow-up appointment because she feared that she will be told off.

She still gets joint pains, and the skin rashes come and go. For the last week, her face has been puffy in the mornings and her legs have been swollen. She is not passing much water, and whatever little that she is passing looks really dark. She had some tests this morning, but no one has so far told her what the problem is.

Her presentation suggests acute nephritis on the background of her SLE. You should use the time to tell her that (1) her presentation is most likely due to lupus nephritis; (2) you would recommend fluid restriction, diuretics, and anti-hypertensives; (3) you will refer her to a nephrologist, who is likely to recommend a renal biopsy; (4) if lupus nephritis is confirmed, the nephrologist will recommend high-dose steroids and stronger immunosuppressive agents; and (5) it is vital to adequately control the inflammation to reduce the risk of permanent renal damage.

During the course of the consultation, you should anticipate some resistance from her when you suggest high-dose steroids because of her concerns about weight gain. Her misconception that the disease might go away should be addressed sympathetically and corrected. You should also reassure her that the team will work with her in partnership and not adopt a paternalistic approach, as she fears being told off for not following their advice.

- Tell her that *her presentation is in keeping with acute nephritis, most likely related to the SLE.*

  'Let me explain what the problem is. If I am going too fast or there is anything you don't understand, please feel free to stop me. At the time when you saw the rheumatologist six months ago with the joint pains and skin rashes, your immune system was attacking your joints and skin. I suspect it is now attacking your kidneys as well.

  'Our kidneys have tiny filters that help produce urine and get rid of the wastes and excess fluid from the body. When the immune system attacks the kidneys, these filters get inflamed. When the filters become inflamed, they are unable to produce enough urine. This is the reason you are not passing enough water. [Pause.] When you don't pass enough water, the wastes and excess fluid start to accumulate in the body. Your legs and face are swollen because of the excess fluid that is accumulating in the body. Your test results show that your kidneys are not clearing the wastes efficiently. [Pause.]

  'Our filters normally do not allow protein or blood to be passed in the urine. We found some protein and blood in your urine, so this again points to inflammation of the kidneys. [Pause.] When the filters become inflamed, the kidneys make a hormone in an attempt to increase the production of urine. This hormone increases the blood pressure. Our blood pressure should normally be less than 130 by 80, but your reading just now was 150 by 100. [Pause.] The rest of your blood tests, the scan of your tummy, and the X-ray of your chest are all normal.'

She says that although she knew that SLE can affect the organs in the body, she never expected that to happen to her. She asks if kidney inflammation is dangerous.

- *Tell her about the short-term complications of acute nephritis and how you will manage them.*

  'The inflammation could potentially worsen and become dangerous, but thankfully, it only happens in a small number of people. We'll continue to keep a close eye on you and take the necessary steps to quickly bring the inflammation under control. If the inflammation worsens, it'll further reduce the ability of the kidneys to get rid of the excess fluid and wastes from the body. The excess fluid could collect in the lungs and make you breathless. The wastes that are not removed can make you feel sick or confused. There is also a risk of the blood pressure rising further and causing some problems.

  'We'll give you a medication through your vein to remove the excess fluid, and another one in the form of a tablet to reduce your blood pressure. I would suggest restricting the amount of fluid that you drink to less than a litre per day, to prevent the accumulation of excess fluid. If the wastes continue to accumulate, you may need a temporary procedure called dialysis to remove the excess fluid and wastes.'

- Tell her that *the risk of developing end-stage kidney disease can be greatly reduced if the inflammation is controlled well*.

  'Apart from removing the excess fluid and reducing the blood pressure, it is important to quickly bring the underlying inflammation under control. If the inflammation is not controlled well, it can lead to permanent damage to the kidneys, requiring long-term dialysis or kidney transplantation. If we control the inflammation well, it'll greatly reduce the risk of damage to the kidneys. The good news is that we have very effective treatments to control the inflammation.'

She asks about the treatments that are used to control the underlying inflammation and if there are any side effects associated with them.

- Tell her that *you will refer her to a nephrologist, who is likely to recommend a renal biopsy*.

  'I'll ask the kidney doctor to see you. Before starting you on treatments to control the underlying inflammation, they are likely to recommend a biopsy. It's a procedure to take a small sample of cells from the kidney using a special needle so that it can be looked under a microscope. It is usually performed by an X-ray doctor, who will use a scanning machine to guide the needle to the correct site. They'll inject a local anaesthetic medicine so that you don't feel any pain from the needle insertion.

  'The biopsy will confirm the inflammation and tell us how bad it is. Some people have more inflammation and a higher chance of damage to the kidneys than others. The kidney doctor will use stronger medicines if the biopsy shows that your inflammation is severe and the risk of long-term damage is greater.'

She asks if there are any complications with a renal biopsy and if she must definitely undergo the procedure.

- *Briefly discuss the complications of a renal biopsy and the disadvantages of not doing one.*

'The kidney doctor will explain the complications before getting your consent to proceed with the biopsy. There is a very small chance of the needle hitting a blood vessel and causing bleeding. The procedure could potentially introduce an infection, but they'll take the necessary precautions to reduce the risk. The doctor performing the procedure will wear a gown and gloves, and clean the area thoroughly before introducing the needle. There is also a small chance that an adequate sample of cells may not be obtained in which case we won't get the information that we need.

'If we don't do the biopsy, we'll have to treat you blindly based on your symptoms and the results of the blood and urine tests. We'll be treating you without the knowledge of the extent of inflammation or damage in the kidneys. We'll, however, respect your wishes if you decide not to undergo the biopsy.'

She asks what treatments will be used to control the underlying inflammation.

- Tell her that *she is likely to be commenced on high-dose steroids and immunosuppressive medications.*

'The kidney doctor is likely to recommend steroids, possibly even before the biopsy is done. They will recommend a much higher dose of steroids than what your rheumatologist suggested to control your joint pain. People who take steroids do put on weight, and there are also other side effects, like a rise in blood pressure, high blood sugar, and thinning of the bones, but we always balance the benefits and risks before starting the treatment. There is a higher chance of permanent damage to the kidneys and ending up on long-term dialysis if the inflammation is not adequately controlled at this stage. I therefore feel that the benefits of steroids far outweigh the risks for you.

'Along with the steroids, the kidney doctor will recommend other medications to calm your immune system once the results of the biopsy are out in a few days. These medications will help quickly taper off the dose of steroids. The kidney doctor will explain all this in detail.'

End the conversation by telling her you will refer her to the nephrologist, who is likely to recommend a renal biopsy and start her on high-dose steroids. Once the results of the biopsy are out, the nephrologist will choose an appropriate immunosuppressive treatment. You would recommend fluid restriction and start her on diuretics and an anti-hypertensive medication in the meantime. Tell her that you will be happy to come back and talk to her if she has any more questions or concerns.

SUMMARY

This scenario tests your skills in discussing an acute complication of a chronic disease. You will be expected to:

- Tell her in layman's terms that her presentation is most likely due to lupus nephritis.
- Discuss the complications of acute nephritis and how you will manage them.

- Tell her that the risk of progression to end-stage kidney disease can be greatly reduced by controlling her inflammation well.
- Briefly discuss the pros and cons of a renal biopsy.
- Tell her that the nephrologist is likely to recommend high-dose steroids and immunosuppressive agents once the diagnosis is confirmed.
- Give her the impression that you will work in partnership with her and not adopt a paternalistic approach.

Capacity, Consent, and Confidentiality

Case 17

The 19-Year-Old Girl Whose Father Objects to a Lumbar Puncture

This 19-year-old Asian girl, a nursing student, was brought to the acute medical unit (AMU) by her parents a couple of hours ago, which was just after 7:00 p.m., with a one-day history of fever, headache, and altered mental state. She was restless and agitated at the time of arrival but calmed down after a small dose of intramuscular haloperidol. Her temperature was 38.2°C, oxygen saturation 98% on room air, pulse rate 88/minute, blood pressure 128/86 mmHg, and respiratory rate 16/minute.

Her parents reported that although she had been unwell since yesterday, with fever and headache, she started behaving strangely and talking gibberish only this morning. There was no trauma to her head, and they did not witness any seizure. She was previously healthy, with no known medical or psychiatric illness. She was not taking any regular medication. She did not smoke, drink alcohol, or use recreational drugs. The date of her last menstrual period was not known.

Physical examination did not reveal any signs of meningism, focal neurological deficits, or skin rash. A non-contrast computed tomography (CT) scan of the brain was normal. Her blood tests showed elevated white cell count of 13.8 × 10⁹/L, but the rest of the blood counts; liver, renal, and thyroid function; coagulation screen; C-reactive protein; urinalysis; and COVID-19 tests were normal. Urine pregnancy test was negative. A portable chest X-ray was normal. Blood samples were sent for culture, and a urine sample was stored for toxicology analysis. She was given a dose of ceftriaxone and dexamethasone an hour ago, and the plan was to start acyclovir after performing a lumbar puncture.

The junior doctor in the AMU, however, tells you that the father has objected to the lumbar puncture and asked to speak to a 'senior doctor'. You are the medical registrar on call. Your task is to talk to the father and address his concerns.

- Introduce yourself and confirm his relationship to the patient. Ask what he has been told already. Do not start the conversation by asking why he is objecting to the lumbar puncture.

He says no one has so far clearly told them what the problem is. The first doctor straightaway assumed that she had a mental illness and asked a lot of questions related to that. The second one, who spent less than a couple of minutes, simply told them that the brain scan was normal and they must do more tests. The one who last spoke to them wanted to do a procedure to collect some fluid from the back to rule out an infection of the brain. He says he would appreciate if you could clearly tell them what the problem is.

After apologising on behalf of the team for not communicating clearly:

- Tell him that *her presentation suggests encephalitis*.

    'We suspect she has a brain infection. This is most likely due to a virus. There are a number of medical conditions that can make a person confused or behave differently, but we suspect it's a brain infection because of the fever and headache.'

- *Discuss the results of the tests done so far.*

    'We did various tests to find out the cause of her illness. The brain scan is normal. A normal brain scan will, however, not rule out an infection. It simply means that there is no bleeding, a large tumour, or pus collection in the brain. The blood tests show that her white blood cells are increased in number. A high white blood cell count is often caused by an infection, but it doesn't tell us where the infection is. Her liver, kidney, and thyroid tests, chest X-ray, and urine tests are all normal. We have sent off a blood sample to check for bacteria, but it'll take at least two days to get that result back.'

He asks if it is serious and how you are treating her.

- Tell him that *you are hoping that she will respond to the treatments*.

    'We have started her on an antibiotic to cover for possible bacterial infection and a steroid medication to reduce the swelling of the brain. We'll stop the antibiotic if we find no evidence of a bacterial infection. We also plan to start her on a medication to treat a common virus that causes brain infection.
    'A brain infection could become serious, but we are hoping that she will respond to these treatments and get better soon. I am unable to say at present how long that would take.'

He wonders how she caught this virus.

- Tell him that herpes simplex virus usually travels from the trigeminal nerve to the brain.

    'The virus that I am referring to is called herpes. It lives in a nerve behind the nose. In some people, it travels from there to the brain and causes brain infection. We do not exactly know why this happens.'

He asks why the other doctor suggested the procedure to remove the fluid from the back, as you seem to have done numerous tests already and started her on antibiotics.

- *Explain why you would like to do a lumbar puncture.*

    'The procedure is done to collect a small amount of the fluid that surrounds the brain and spinal cord. We call it lumbar puncture. We'll place a needle in the space between the bones in the lower part of the back to collect the fluid. We'll inject an anaesthetic *medicine locally so that she doesn't feel any pain. It should take less than 15 minutes to do this procedure.*

'*The treatments that we are giving her now are based on our knowledge of the most common bugs that cause brain infection. Testing the fluid will help us identify the bacteria or virus that is causing the infection and find out if we are on the right track with the treatments that we have started. If we find an infection different to what we are suspecting, we will modify the treatment accordingly.*'

- Tell him that *there are no alternative tests* that can provide the same information.

'*The information that we get by testing the fluid cannot be obtained by any other means. Brain scans or X-rays cannot identify the bug that is causing the brain infection. We have sent off her blood sample to check for bacteria in her blood, but it may or may not be helpful. Moreover, it will not show the viruses. Testing the fluid is the only way to make an accurate diagnosis.*'

He says he is not happy for you to do the procedure. When asked for the reason, he says he discussed this with his sister. She told him that the procedure is dangerous and it can cause paralysis of the legs.

- *Reassure him that lumbar puncture does not cause paralysis.*

'*That is not true. The procedure does not cause paralysis. The needle is inserted well below the point where the spinal cord ends, so there is no chance of spinal cord or nerve damage.*'

- *Tell him about the risks of the procedure.*

'*The risks of the procedure are very small compared to the dangers of not making a correct diagnosis. About one in three people may get a headache after this procedure. We use a smaller needle to minimise this risk. If she gets a headache, we'll make sure she's given enough fluids and painkillers. It usually resolves within a few days.*'

'*Some people get a backache which may shoot down the leg. If we accidentally poke a small blood vessel when we insert the needle, there may be some bleeding. There is a very small risk of introducing an infection, but we'll take great care to clean the skin thoroughly before we insert the needle. In people with a high pressure in the brain, removing the fluid can cause a downward movement of the brain. However, it is extremely unlikely in her, as the brain scan has ruled out a high pressure in her brain.*'

- Warn him that *it is possible that you may not be able to obtain any fluid.*

'*There is a small chance that we may not get any fluid. If we can't get any fluid, we'll ask an anaesthetic doctor to do the procedure. Hopefully, that won't be necessary.*'

- *You will perform the procedure yourself.*

'*I'll perform the procedure myself instead of asking a junior colleague to do it. I have done a number of lumbar punctures. I will take great care to ensure that it all goes well.*'

Consent must be obtained from all adults (with some exceptions) before healthcare interventions, including physical examination, investigations, procedures, treatments, and specialist referrals. It may be implied, verbal, or written. All patients, including those with intellectual disability, have a legal right to autonomy. There are three requirements for consent to be valid:

1. The person from whom consent is obtained must have *mental capacity*.
2. The person must be *provided with as much information as possible* so that it is an informed consent.
3. The decision must be *voluntary* and not coerced.

Assessment of capacity is a two-step process:

1. The first step is to check if there is an impairment of the mind or brain (e.g. dementia, mental illness, encephalitis, intoxication).
2. If an impairment of the mind or brain is not identified, the second step is to establish if the person is able to understand the information, retain the information for long enough, weigh the pros and cons, and communicate the decision.

Those who are unable to do any of these are deemed to not have decision-making capacity.

All adults (>18 years of age in the UK) must be assumed to have capacity unless it can be established otherwise. Children can provide consent if they are 'Gillick competent' (have sufficient intelligence and maturity to understand the nature of the intervention). Capacity is decision-specific. The question is whether the person is able to make a specific decision at a specific point in time, not whether they have the capacity to make decisions generally. For example, a person may be able to consent to blood taking but not to major abdominal surgery. A person with capacity can decline the intervention even if it is life-saving (e.g. refusal of blood transfusion by a Jehovah's Witness). The informed refusal of consent by a person with capacity cannot be overridden, however irrational, and the doctor who treats a person against their wishes can be sued for battery. Family members cannot consent on behalf of an adult who has capacity. Loss of capacity may be temporary (e.g. encephalitis, alcohol intoxication) or fluctuate during the course of the day. In difficult cases, you should seek expert help to assess the capacity (e.g. psychiatrist). If the difficulty is due to language or cultural barrier, you should seek the help of a qualified interpreter or a cultural support person.

If the person lacks capacity, treatment can be provided lawfully in the following situations:

1. In the best interests of the person in an emergency setting. Best interest is decided on the basis of the treatment that would give the best possible outcome, taking into consideration the known values, beliefs, or preferences of the person lacking capacity.
2. If the person has appointed a lasting power of attorney.
3. If a court has appointed a deputy to act on behalf of the person.
4. Under the Mental Health Act (MHA).

It is important to note that MHA only authorises the treatment of the mental disorder and *not* the physical illness. Treatment of the physical illness should still take the person's best interests into consideration.

In this case, consent is *not* required from the father to perform the lumbar puncture. It can be performed in her best interests. However, in practice, it won't be easy to get past the father and forcefully perform the procedure on her. It is difficult to tell him that we do not need his consent or that the medical team would like to proceed taking into account her best interests. Moreover, families decide on behalf of the patient in many parts of the world. Surveys have shown that a large proportion of parents in some countries refuse lumbar puncture for their children because they believe that the procedure is risky.

An exception can be made when life-saving treatments are refused by a family member for a patient without capacity (e.g. emergency dialysis for a patient with life-threatening acute kidney injury). The case can then be discussed with the most senior member of the clinical team (e.g. medical director) and a court order sought to forcefully treat the patient.

He says he will discuss with his family members and let you know his decision.

Tell him that:

- *The benefits of lumbar puncture far outweigh the risks.*

    'I'd like to reassure you once again that lumbar puncture is generally a very safe procedure. The benefits of the procedure far outweigh the risks. Infection of the brain can lead to serious consequences if it is not treated correctly. Your daughter is very unwell. We want her to get well soon.

    'It is important to know if we are giving her the correct treatments. The treatments that we have started may or may not work. If we don't perform the procedure, we won't know how to proceed further in case she doesn't respond to the current treatments. I am sorry if you feel that I am rushing you, but we must take a decision soon. If we delay the lumbar puncture, the results may not be accurate, as she would have received the antibiotics for quite a while by then. The scans and blood tests cannot give us this information.'

If he remains unconvinced, do not accede to his demands but end the conversation by telling him that you will ask a more senior colleague (e.g. intensive care unit or AMU consultant, depending on who is available at that time) to talk to him.

SUMMARY

This scenario tests your skills in convincing a difficult father before performing a procedure on his young daughter. You will be expected to:

- Clearly explain the suspected diagnosis and the results of the tests in layman's terms.
- Explain why you are recommending a lumbar puncture.
- Explore the reasons if he objects to the procedure.
- Allay his anxieties about the risk of paralysis with lumbar puncture.
- Offer a second opinion if he is still not convinced.

Not managing to convince him will not lead to an unsatisfactory mark, as long as you tell him the correct things and end the conversation by offering to get your senior to come and talk to him instead of acceding. This is different from directly talking to a patient to obtain consent to perform a procedure or start a new medication. If the patient refuses, you must respect their wishes, as long as (1) they are deemed to have capacity, (2) you have provided enough information for them to make an informed decision, and (3) you are convinced that their decision is voluntary and not coerced.

A variation of this case is seeking consent for a lumbar puncture from a patient with suspected subarachnoid haemorrhage and normal CT scan result.

The 66-Year-Old Man Who Does Not Wish to Start Dialysis

This 66-year-old retired immigration officer with a background history of end-stage kidney disease, diabetes mellitus, hypertension, and hyperlipidaemia presented to the acute medical unit (AMU) yesterday with acute worsening of his chronic breathlessness. He denied other cardiorespiratory symptoms. His regular medications included insulin, glipizide, valsartan, amlodipine, atorvastatin, furosemide, erythropoietin, multivitamins, calcium acetate, and alfacalcidol.

On examination, he was found to have features of fluid overload, with satisfactory oxygen saturation. His haemoglobin was 88 g/L, serum creatinine 878 μmol/L, and estimated glomerular filtration rate <15 mL/min. His echocardiogram done some months ago showed an ejection fraction of 55%.

Following strict fluid restriction and intravenous diuretics, his symptoms have somewhat improved. The AMU consultant feels that he must start dialysis as soon as possible via a permcath. Of note, he was advised by his renal consultant several months ago to consider haemodialysis and get an arteriovenous fistula created, but he wanted time to think about it. You are the medical registrar in the AMU. Your task is to discuss this with him.

- Introduce yourself, and confirm his identity. Ask how he is and what he has been told about his kidney disease.

He says he is feeling better. He knows that his kidney problem is quite advanced. For the last year, he has been getting tired very easily and out of breath on exertion. The kidney doctor recommended dialysis and asked him to go for a small operation on his forearm, but he has been reluctant.

- Tell him that *his breathlessness was caused by fluid overload* secondary to advanced chronic kidney disease.

'I am sorry to hear that your health has been declining. Your kidney problem is indeed quite advanced. The damaged kidneys are not able to efficiently get rid of the excess fluid, wastes, and toxins from your body. You felt more breathless yesterday because of the collection of excess fluid in your lungs.

'We gave you the water tablet in the form of an injection to remove the excess fluid. I am glad to hear that this treatment has worked and you are feeling better now. I'd recommend continuing the water tablet and restricting the amount of fluid that you drink in a day to prevent the build-up of excess fluid.'

- Ask what he understands about dialysis and what exactly his concerns are.

He says he was told that he must go to a dialysis centre three times a week to be connected to a machine that cleans the blood. He has been reluctant because he didn't like the idea of being strapped to a machine three times a week. He doesn't wish to live his life like that.

Tell him that:

- **You would recommend commencing dialysis as soon as possible.**

'I hear you. I am sorry if you think I am pressuring you, but we must take a decision soon, as your kidney function is much worse now. Without dialysis, I'm afraid you could die soon, possibly within months. Dialysis will help to not only significantly prolong your life but also reduce your tiredness and breathing trouble. It'll improve your overall quality of life. Apart from getting a kidney transplant, for which there is a very long wait, dialysis is the only definitive way to remove the excess fluid, wastes, and toxins from your body. It is not possible to do this by giving you medicines alone.'

- **Dialysis must be commenced via a permcath**, as an arteriovenous fistula (AVF) will take time to mature.

'The small operation that your kidney doctor recommended is to join an artery and a vein – the two types of blood vessels in our body – in your forearm to create a connection. We call this a fistula. The fistula will be used to draw blood from your body and then return it back after running it through a dialysis machine.

'It'll take several weeks, however, before we can start using the fistula for dialysis, as its lining needs to get harder. We cannot wait that long, so we must temporarily place a soft plastic tube in a large blood vessel in your neck to start dialysis straightaway. There are two bores in this tube – one to draw blood from your body and the other to return the blood after cleaning it. The tube will be hanging down from your chest. We'll remove this tube once the fistula is ready to be used for dialysis.'

He asks if dialysis is absolutely safe. With all his medical conditions, he wonders if the benefits of dialysis really outweigh the risks.

Tell him that:

- **There are no contraindications to starting dialysis.**

'We discourage dialysis in people who have too many medical problems, as there may not be much to be gained. However, in your case, we feel that the benefits of dialysis far outweigh the risks. Diabetes, high blood pressure, and high cholesterol are, in fact, quite common among people with kidney disease.'

- *There are some complications associated with dialysis and the use of permcath.*

'There are, indeed, some risks associated with dialysis. When you first start dialysis, you may experience symptoms like dizziness, cramping of the muscles, tiredness, and exhaustion, but they should pass after the first few sessions. Additionally, there are some problems with the placement of the tube in the neck. It can become blocked or infected – we may have to change the tube if this happens. If the tube gets infected, you will be admitted to the hospital and given a prolonged course of antibiotics. While the tube is being placed, there is a risk of bleeding or accidentally poking the layer around the lung – this can cause air to collect around the lung. The doctor who places the tube will explain these risks to you before getting your consent to proceed.'

He asks if he can stop his medications if he starts dialysis.

- Tell him that *dialysis cannot replicate all the functions of the kidneys.*

'Apart from clearing the wastes from the body, the kidneys also produce a few hormones – one of them helps us produce the blood cells, and another one makes vitamin D work.
'When the kidneys get damaged, they stop producing these hormones. Dialysis only helps clear the wastes. It cannot restore the production of these hormones. You should therefore continue the medicine that you inject beneath the skin – this will help you make the blood cells – and the vitamin D tablet. You should also continue taking the medications for your diabetes, blood pressure, and high cholesterol.'

He says he appreciates your explanation but he is not keen to start dialysis.

- *Explore the reasons for the refusal.*

Refusal of consent may be due to financial concerns (in countries where health service is not free), fear of side effects or complications, misunderstanding of the intended benefits, or misinformation (e.g. he may know someone who had a bad experience with dialysis).

- *Check his understanding* of the information that was provided.

It is important to check his understanding, because his refusal of consent is valid only if we are convinced that he has *capacity* and he is *voluntarily* making an *informed decision*. It is particularly important for him to understand that his lifespan will be significantly shortened without dialysis.

He says he has had a fulfilling life. Although he has had the high blood pressure and diabetes for many years, he did not have any symptoms until a year ago. He understands that dialysis can prolong his life and improve his tiredness and breathing trouble, but that is not how he wishes to live his life. He would rather remain independent for the remainder of his life, even if it is only for a few months.

- Tell him that *you will offer more time.* Encourage him to discuss with his family and friends.

'I agree that going for dialysis three times a week is like doing a part-time job. It is a tough decision, indeed. We will, of course, respect your wishes. However, please take

some more time and discuss with your family or friends to see what they think. I'll give
you some written information to go through and let the kidney doctors know about your
decision. I am sure the kidney doctor can arrange for you to be taken around a dialysis
unit and speak to some patients, if you wish.'

He says he will take up your suggestion and speak to his wife. He asks how he will be managed if he does not commence dialysis.

Tell him that:

- **Palliative measures will be instituted if he is not keen on dialysis.**

  'If you are not keen to start dialysis, we'll seek the help of the palliative doctors. They
  are experts on providing treatments that relieve suffering and improve the quality of life.
  This is particularly important because your symptoms may get worse as the wastes and
  toxins continue to build up in the body. Palliative treatments will aim to improve symp-
  toms like tiredness, breathing trouble, itching, and sickness.'

- **He can change his mind later.**

  'If you change your mind later, please let us know. There are also people who change
  their mind after starting dialysis and ask for it to be withdrawn.'

Advance care planning (ACP) may be broached with patients with chronic kidney disease, especially those who refuse dialysis, but it may not be the right time to bring up this topic, as you have given him some more time to think about dialysis and he has agreed to discuss this with his wife. The ACP discussion can take place once we know for sure that he is firm in his decision.

SUMMARY

This scenario tests your skills in communicating with a patient who is refusing a life-sustaining treatment. You will be expected to:

- Explain that his breathlessness was caused by fluid overload.
- Provide information about dialysis, including the benefits, risks, and alternatives.
- If the patient refuses the proposed intervention, explore the reasons for refusal.
- Check his decision-making capacity, and ensure that his decision is voluntary and not coerced.
- Give him more time, and suggest discussing with family members or friends.
- Tell him that you will respect his wishes but he can let you know if he changes his mind later.

A variation of this case is talking to a Jehovah's Witness who is refusing blood transfusion after being admitted with massive upper gastrointestinal bleeding. You will be expected to:

- Explain the possible cause of her bleeding and the seriousness of her condition.
- Provide the necessary information, including the benefits of blood transfusion, consequences of not receiving the transfusion (which may include death), risks of transfusion, and alternative treatments (e.g. measures to stop the bleeding, fluids to improve blood pressure).
- Assess her decision-making capacity if she refuses transfusion.

If she insists on not receiving any blood products after hearing the information, you should make sure that her decision is voluntary and not coerced. Her decision may be irrational and incomprehensible, but we must respect her autonomy. The decision should be to withhold the transfusion, even if it means that she will die without the blood transfusion. Her case should be discussed with the senior-most clinician and the clinical ethics team. The details of all the conversations should be documented.

The 33-Year-Old Man Who Is Refusing the HIV Test

This 33-year-old man, a professional guitarist, was admitted to the high-dependency unit (HDU) four days ago with a four-day history of fever, dry cough, and breathlessness. His past medical history is unremarkable. He does not take any regular medication. He smokes about ten cigarettes a day and drinks two cans of beer on most days. He told the admitting doctor that he is single.

His vital signs at the time of admission showed tachycardia, tachypnoea, and low oxygen saturation by pulse oximetry. His lungs were clear. The rest of the examination was unremarkable. Arterial blood gases showed hypoxaemia.

His blood tests revealed elevated white cell count and C-reactive protein of 28 mg/dl, but the rest of the blood counts and liver and renal functions were normal. Chest X-ray showed perihilar fluffy shadows. His blood cultures were sterile, but silver staining of his induced sputum sample was reported as positive for *Pneumocystis jirovecii* and negative for acid-fast bacilli. He was initially commenced on amoxicillin–clavulanic acid and then switched to high-dose co-trimoxazole after the sputum results became available two days ago.

He has clinically improved since admission. His vital signs are now normal, and he has been off oxygen for more than 24 hours. You are the registrar covering his ward. You have not met him before, as he was transferred from the HDU to your ward only last night. Your task is to ask for his consent to test him for human immunodeficiency virus (HIV).

- Introduce yourself, and confirm his identity. Ask if he is feeling better and what he has been told so far about his illness.

He says he is feeling a lot better now compared to how he was four days ago. He is coughing less, and his breathing is much better. He says the ICU doctor told him that his X-ray showed a lung infection and some bug was found in his phlegm sample. He knows that he is getting antibiotics to treat the infection.

DOI: 10.1201/9781003533337-22

Tell him that:

- *His sputum result is positive for* Pneumocystis jirovecii, *which suggests that he may be immunocompromised.*

'Your phlegm test shows that your lung infection is caused by a bug called Pneumocystis. This infection usually occurs in people with weak immunity. It is not seen in people with a healthy immune system.'

- *HIV infection is one of the causes of an immunocompromised state.*

'There are a few possible causes for weak immunity. One is being born with a weak immune system due to a faulty gene. I think that is unlikely in your case, as you would have had repeated infections dating from your childhood days and not be presenting to us for the first time at the age of 33. The second is taking medications that suppress the immune system, which you don't seem to be. The third is HIV infection. What do you know about HIV?'

He says he knows that HIV is transmitted by sexual intercourse.

- Ask if he has ever been tested for HIV infection.
- *Check for risk factors for HIV.* Start with:

'Would you mind if I ask you some sensitive questions to check if you are at risk of getting HIV?'

Ask how long he has been single and if he has had any sexual partners in the past. Were they male or female? How many partners has he had? If he is gay, is he the receiving or inserting partner? Was the intercourse protected or unprotected? Does he know if any of them was HIV-positive? When was the last time he had intercourse? Has he ever visited sex workers? Has he ever shared needles, had tattoos with unsterile needles, or received a blood transfusion?

He says he has never had an HIV test. He has been single since splitting up with his boyfriend about three months ago. He has been gay all his life. He has had multiple casual sexual partners since he was 18 years old. He is usually the receiving partner. The intercourse has always been unprotected. He is not sure if his partners have been tested for HIV. He has never visited commercial sex workers. He has never injected drugs, had tattoos, or received a blood transfusion.

- Tell him that that *you would recommend an HIV test.*

'I wonder if your lowered immunity is caused by HIV. HIV is a virus that is transmitted by infected body fluids during sexual intercourse. It is more common among men who have sex with men. Based on what you have told me, I would strongly recommend doing an HIV test. Can I discuss this further?'

He says he does not wish to be tested for HIV.

Patients who refuse an HIV test often do so because of incorrect beliefs about the infection or the negative consequences of getting a positive result. There may be fear of stigmatisation and discrimination. He has the right to decline the test, but his reasons for refusal should be explored, and the benefits of testing clearly explained to him.

There are several benefits in getting tested:

1. Effective medications are available to treat HIV infection and prevent progression to acquired immunodeficiency syndrome (AIDS).
2. In patients with AIDS, treatment will result in a rise in the CD4 count and a reduction of the risk of further opportunistic infections.
3. The life expectancy of those with AIDS could be extended by several years.
4. If the viral load is undetectable, there is no risk of transmission to sexual partners.
5. Knowing the HIV status will reduce anxiety.

He says he does not wish to carry that label for the rest of his life. He feels that his work colleagues and friends will start to view him differently if they find out that he is HIV-positive.

Tell him that:

- **The test result is confidential** and will only be shared with him.

  'The result will only be shared with you. You don't have to disclose the result to your employer or work colleagues. We have come a long way, and it is not like how it used to be about 20–30 years ago. Employers are not supposed to discriminate anyone on the basis of a positive HIV test result. You can even take legal action against those who do.'

- **He has a right to decline the test**, but you would like to explain the benefits of getting tested.

  'You, of course, have the right to decline the test, but I would strongly encourage you to get tested. Please allow me to explain the benefits of getting tested.'

- If he is found to be HIV-positive, **effective treatments are available**.

  'The virus that causes HIV infection destroys a type of white blood cell called CD4 that protects us from infection – this lowers the immunity and increases the risk of getting some unusual infections that generally do not occur in people with healthy immunity. Once the immunity is lowered because of HIV, we call it AIDS – it is an acronym for acquired immunodeficiency syndrome. It is called acquired as it is not present at birth, and immunodeficiency is the medical term for weak immunity.

  'If you are found to have HIV, it means that it has already progressed to AIDS, as we have found this unusual infection in your lung. You are at risk of getting further unusual infections, but the good news is that we have very good treatments for HIV. By reducing the amount of virus in the blood, these treatments will help stop the destruction of the white blood cells and greatly reduce the risk of getting these infections.'

- *Treatment of HIV can help extend the lifespan of those with AIDS* by several years.

'Once HIV infection progresses to AIDS, I am afraid it could significantly shorten the lifespan. The treatments for HIV have been shown to prolong the lifespan by several years. We already have very effective treatments for HIV, but at the pace at which research is being conducted in this field, the treatments are only likely to get better and better in the coming years.'

- *Treatment of HIV will help reduce the risk of transmission to others.*

'If we manage to bring the amount of virus in the blood to an undetectable level with treatment, you will not be passing the virus to your future sexual partners.'

He asks if he should tell his ex-partners if his result comes back as positive.

Partner notification is a key component of HIV counselling. If his result comes back positive, he should be encouraged to disclose it to his sexual partners so that they, too, could be tested and commenced on treatment, if necessary. Many patients will be reluctant to do so, thus posing a legal, ethical, and moral challenge for clinicians. It creates a conflict between autonomy and respect for confidentiality versus protecting the health of the sexual partner(s) at risk.

He should also be made aware of the legal position regarding disclosure, which varies in different parts of the world. In the UK, there is no legal obligation for an HIV-positive individual to disclose the result to his sexual partner, but it will become a criminal offence if he knowingly transmits HIV to someone. He could be prosecuted if it is proved that (1) he knew that he was HIV-positive and had a detectable viral load, (2) he engaged in unprotected intercourse without telling the partner about his HIV status, and (3) the partner acquired HIV as a result.

Tell him that:

- *You would encourage him to disclose it to his sexual partners.*

'Yes, we would encourage you to disclose it to your ex-partners, so that they, too, can be tested and started on treatment if they test positive.'

- *He does not have to always disclose to his future sexual partners.*

'You do not have to tell your future sexual partners as long as you are on treatment, there is no virus in your blood, and you use a condom.'

- *He could be prosecuted if he recklessly transmits HIV to someone.*

'However, you should bear in mind that it will become a criminal offence if you knowingly transmit HIV to your partner. If it is proved in court that you had unprotected intercourse with your partner without telling him about your HIV result, you could be prosecuted. You won't be charged if you use a condom and there is no virus in your blood.'

End the conversation by telling him that once he has made up his mind, you will arrange for him to have the test. Tell him that the result should be available within three days. If the result is positive, he will be referred to an HIV specialist so that he can be started on appropriate treatment and closely monitored.

SUMMARY

This scenario tests your skills in convincing a patient with high-risk behaviour and *Pneumocystis* infection to get tested for HIV. You will be expected to:

- Tell him that his pneumonia is caused by an opportunistic infection.
- Explain why you are recommending an HIV test.
- Check for the presence of risk factors for HIV.
- Tell him that he has a right to decline the test.
- Explain the benefits of getting tested (e.g. prevention of opportunistic infection, prolonged life expectancy, reduced risk of transmission to sexual partners, elimination of anxiety).
- Reassure him that the test result is confidential and will only be shared with him.
- Discuss the issues around partner notification, and warn him about the legal requirements.

The 52-Year-Old Man Who Wants to Get Discharged against Medical Advice

This 52-year-old man with a background history of hyperlipidaemia and impaired glucose tolerance was admitted last night with acute central chest pain. He was diagnosed with non–ST elevation acute coronary syndrome (NSTE-ACS) on the basis of elevated high-sensitivity troponin and normal 12-lead electrocardiogram (ECG) at the time of admission. He had a further episode of chest pain after admission when the ECG showed ST segment depression.

Because of the dynamic ECG changes, the cardiologist has arranged to perform an invasive coronary angiogram later this morning. He has already been commenced on dual anti-platelet therapy, low-molecular-weight heparin, nitrates, and high-dose statin. His vital signs are all normal.

The nurse asks if you could speak to him as he told her that he does not wish to stay in the hospital anymore. You are the medical registrar on call.

Introduce yourself, and confirm his identity. Tell him that you have come to talk to him as you heard from the nurse that he wishes to get discharged.

- Ask if he is well, and *find out why he wants to go home*.

He says the pain has gone and he feels well. He has not had any chest pain for more than eight hours. He says he is grateful to the team and appreciates their care, but he doesn't think he needs to stay in the hospital anymore. He wants to get discharged as soon as possible. He says he is an estate agent and has a few important appointments later that day, which he cannot afford to miss.

This man wants to leave the hospital against medical advice (AMA) even before the completion of his workup or treatment. This is different from abscondment, where the patient decides to leave the hospital without letting anyone know. Patients ask to leave AMA either because (1) they feel better, (2) they are unhappy with the care, (3) they do not clearly understand the reasons for having to stay in the hospital, or (4) they have obligations at home or at work.

The patient must have mental capacity to leave AMA. Patients with mental capacity have the right to refuse the interventions suggested by the healthcare provider, including those that are life-sustaining. Those with altered mental state (e.g. intoxication, psychosis, dementia) who wish to leave AMA may pose a challenge, however. If in doubt, the mental capacity should be formally assessed, and the help of a psychiatrist sought.

The dynamic ECG changes in this man suggest ongoing cardiac ischaemia. He clearly needs close monitoring in the inpatient setting, as his condition is unstable and there is a potential threat to his life. Moreover, the treatments planned for him cannot be delivered in the outpatient setting or at home.

- *Ask what he understands about his condition.*

He says he was told that the pain was due to heart problem. He is aware that the consultant wants to do some procedure on his heart. He was half-asleep when the doctor in the ward told him about it, so he is not entirely sure why the consultant wants to do that.

Explain the seriousness of his condition. Tell him that:

- His chest pain was caused by acute myocardial infarction.

  'I am afraid you've had a heart attack. A heart attack occurs when a blood vessel supplying the heart muscle suddenly gets blocked by a blood clot. It stops the blood from flowing through that blood vessel and causes damage to the heart muscle.'

- Myocardial infarction can lead to complications and even death, if not treated promptly.

  'A heart attack can lead to some complications, some of which are serious and potentially life-threatening. The chance of developing these complications depends on how much of the heart muscle is damaged. With a large heart attack, the heart muscle becomes so weak that it cannot pump enough blood around the body. Fluid can build up in the lungs, making it hard to breathe and get enough oxygen. The heartbeat can become dangerously fast and irregular. People who survive a large heart attack may be left with permanent damage to the heart muscle and develop some long-term problems. It is therefore important that we try to restore the blood flow to the heart muscle and limit the damage as much as possible.'

- The dynamic changes on his ECG suggest ongoing ischaemia and risk of extension of the infarct.

  'When you complained of chest pain, we saw some changes on the tracing of your heart. It means the blood flow through the blocked blood vessel hasn't been restored and there is a risk of further damage to the heart muscle.'

He says he is happy to take some pills to treat the heart attack. He just does not want to stay in the hospital. He asks if it is really necessary for him to undergo the procedure.

Explain why he must stay in the hospital. Tell him that:

- He has been commenced on appropriate medications to limit the extension of the infarct.

   'The medicines that we are giving you will help widen the blood vessels that supply the heart, make the blood less sticky, and prevent further blood clots from forming. You do not have any pain now possibly because of these medicines.'

- The cardiologist has recommended the procedure to enable revascularisation.

   'Medicines alone are not enough to limit the damage to the heart muscle. The heart doctor has recommended the procedure to further widen the blocked blood vessel. During this procedure, he will pass a long thin tube through your groin or wrist and advance it into the blood vessels around the heart. With the help of an X-ray machine, he'll place the tube in the narrowed blood vessel. There is a balloon at the tip of the tube, which will be blown up to widen the narrowed blood vessel. We call this angioplasty. A small wire mesh tube called a stent is usually then left in the blood vessel to stop it from closing again.'

- You would strongly recommend staying in the hospital.

   'I would strongly advise you to stay in the hospital, so that we can continue to monitor you closely and give you the necessary treatments. It is vital to open the blocked blood vessel and limit the damage to the heart muscle so that you do not suffer any complications from the heart attack. If all goes well, you should be able to go home in two to three days.'

Pause for a moment and check his understanding before proceeding further.

- *If he says he would still prefer to leave, offer some options.*

   'Do you want me to give you some time to think through what I just told you? Shall I come back and talk to you again a little later?' 'Do you think you can delegate the work to one of your colleagues?' or 'Would you like to discuss this with any of your friends or family members?'

He says he appreciates your concern and the explanation but he would still like to go. He does not need more time. He will lose his commission if he delegates the task to his colleague. He does not wish to discuss with any of his family members. He is divorced, and there isn't anyone close in his family.

You should now *assess his mental capacity*.

- Ask him to tell you what he has understood. You should particularly check if he has fully understood the benefits of staying and the risks of leaving.

He says he understands that he has had a heart attack which is caused by a blood clot blocking a blood vessel supplying the heart. The heart attack can cause more damage to the heart muscle if he doesn't stay in the hospital and get the procedure done. He understands that he could die or develop some long-term complications if the heart attack is not treated properly. He would still prefer to take a chance and leave. He is happy to take the medicines that you have prescribed for the heart attack.

He has mental capacity because he has understood what you told him, retained the information for long enough, weighed the pros and cons, and communicated his decision clearly. He has no impairment of his brain or mind. His autonomy takes precedence over beneficence. His voluntary and informed refusal of consent, although irrational, cannot be overridden. Our job is to provide a professional opinion, not force an adult with capacity to accept all our recommendations.

- Tell him that *you will respect his wishes and allow him to go after he signs a form*. You will prescribe the medications and arrange an outpatient appointment with the cardiologist.

'I'll respect your wishes. You'll have to sign a form before you leave. I'll inform my consultant. I'll also let the heart doctor know that you won't be having the procedure. I hope you won't mind if I ask him to see you in his clinic. I'll arrange for you to receive all the medications except for the blood-thinning medication that we are giving you as an injection in the tummy. Once you are ready, please ask someone to come and pick you. It's not a good idea for you to go alone.'

- Tell him that *he should not hesitate to come back if the chest pain returns*.

'If you change your mind or the chest pain comes back, please do not hesitate to come back. You may have to call an ambulance. I hope you don't mind me saying this, but it is not a good idea to go to work. You should at least rest at home for the next few days and not strain your heart too much.'

It is important to document the discussion you had with him, clearly stating that (1) he decided to leave AMA; (2) you explained the benefits of staying and the risks of leaving, including the potential threat to his life; (3) he had mental capacity and fully understood what you said; (4) you told him that he can return any time; (5) you have arranged follow-up with the cardiologist; and (6) you discussed his case with your consultant and the cardiologist.

SUMMARY

This scenario tests your skills in communicating with a patient who wishes to leave the hospital AMA. You will be expected to:

- Find out why he wants to get discharged against medical advice.
- Check his understanding of the condition.

- Explain the seriousness of his illness and why you would like him to stay in the hospital.
- Tell him that the treatments that have been planned (e.g. coronary angioplasty) cannot be administered in the outpatient setting.
- If he insists on leaving, assess his mental capacity.

Make sure he has clearly understood the benefits of staying in the hospital and the risks of leaving.

- Offer some options depending on his reasons for wanting to leave.
- If he is still not convinced, provide clear instruction on what he must do if the chest pain returns.

A variation of this case is talking to a patient admitted after paracetamol overdose who is asking to leave the hospital. You should explain (1) the risks to the health (e.g. liver damage, kidney injury, and potential risk of death), (2) the treatments that you are administering (e.g. N-acetylcysteine), and (3) why you would recommend staying in the hospital (e.g. the need for close monitoring, risk of further deterioration). If the patient insists on leaving, you must assess her capacity and suicidal risk.

- If she lacks capacity, she can be treated in her best interests.
- If she has capacity but is suicidal, she can be sectioned and detained in the hospital under the 'Mental Health Act' (as she poses a risk of harm to herself) but cannot be treated for the overdose against her wishes unless there is a court order to do so.
- If she has capacity and is not suicidal in the opinion of a psychiatrist, you should provide clear advice on when to return to the hospital (after trying your best to ask her to stay).

Offer outpatient treatment if feasible (e.g. oral methionine and advise her to return on the following day for blood tests), and make sure the case is discussed with the senior-most clinician.

Case 21

The 77-Year-Old Man Whose Daughter Asks You Not to Reveal the Diagnosis of Cancer to Him

This 77-year-old Asian man with a background history of hypertension, diabetes, hyperlipidaemia, and chronic kidney disease stage 3 was admitted a few days ago with a two-week history of cough, shortness of breath on exertion, and loss of appetite. He denied fever, haemoptysis, or weight loss.

Physical examination revealed absent air entry on the left side but was otherwise unremarkable. The chest X-ray showed features in keeping with a large left-sided pleural effusion. His blood test results showed serum creatinine 104 µmol/L, estimated glomerular filtration rate 40 mL/minute, and C-reactive protein 18 mg/dl. The blood counts, liver function tests, serum electrolytes, and calcium were normal. He was empirically commenced on amoxicillin–clavulanic acid.

About 2,000 mL of fluid has been drained from his left pleural cavity over the last four days. The computed tomography (CT) scan of the thorax, abdomen, and pelvis, which was performed after draining the pleural fluid, has been reported as showing a mass-like consolidation in the left lower lobe, with enlarged mediastinal nodes, multiple liver metastases, and compression fracture of the T12 vertebra. His pleural fluid cytology has been reported as positive for thyroid transcription factor-1 (TTF-1), in keeping with adenocarcinoma of the lung. There was no evidence of tuberculosis or bacterial infection in the pleural fluid.

At the time of admission, the patient asked the medical team to discuss all his test results and treatment plan with his family. The family was told that there was fluid around the lung, the possible cause of which was infection or 'something more serious'. Your task is to update his daughter on the results of the CT scan and pleural fluid cytology.

- Introduce yourself, and confirm the identity and the relationship of the daughter. Ask what she has been told already.

The daughter says she was told about the fluid collection around the lung and that this could be due to infection or possibly something more serious. Although the doctors did not tell her what exactly they meant by the word 'serious', she guessed that they were suspecting cancer. She is anxiously waiting to find out the results of the scan and the other tests that were done.

DOI: 10.1201/9781003533337-24

- Tell her that *the test results are in keeping with cancer.*

  '*I am afraid your suspicions are correct. The news is not good. [Pause.] The scan shows cancer.*'

Give her a moment to digest the news before continuing. Then tell her that:

- **The cancer is already in the advanced stage.**

  '*The cancer is quite advanced. It has already spread from the lung to the lymph glands in the centre of the chest and to the liver. There is a broken bone in the middle of his spine, so we suspect the cancer has spread to his backbone as well. I am sorry.*'

The daughter becomes tearful and says she is very disappointed to hear the news. She was hoping that it was only an infection. She asks if you are absolutely certain that it is cancer and not infection.

- Tell her that the pleural fluid cytology was positive for TTF-1, which is in keeping with cancer and not infection.

  '*I wish I had better news for you. We would normally take a sample from the tumour to be examined under a microscope to confirm that it is due to cancer. We don't have to do that for him, however, because we found cancer cells in the fluid that we drained from the space around the lung. Moreover, the scan result showing the spread to the liver and lymph glands is in keeping with cancer, not infection.*'

She asks how he will be treated and how long he can expect to live.

Give her a brief idea of the treatments for lung cancer and his prognosis. Tell her that:

- You will be referring him to a medical oncologist.

  '*We'll be referring him to a cancer specialist, who will discuss the treatment plan.*'

- His cancer cannot be cured.

  '*As his cancer has already spread outside the lung, it cannot be cured. It means we cannot get rid of the cancer. The intent of treatment will be to prolong his life and control the symptoms.*'

- His prognosis depends on various factors.

  '*It's difficult to accurately predict how much time he has left. It largely depends on whether or not he prefers to receive any treatment. Some people with advanced cancer take a conscious decision to not receive any treatment. If he prefers to not receive any treatment, my guess is that he will probably live another six months. If he receives treatment for the cancer, then it depends on how well he responds to it. Some of the new treatments for lung cancer can help prolong life significantly, but there is a chance that they may not work at all or stop working after a while.*'

She recalls her grandmother receiving chemotherapy for blood cancer many years ago and suffering severe side effects. She would rather not choose that option for her father. She asks how he will be managed if they prefer not to accept any treatment.

Discuss the possible treatments for his lung cancer. Tell her that:

- The treatments for lung cancer have vastly advanced.

  'I am sorry to hear about your grandmother. Chemotherapy involves giving medications to stop the cancer cells from multiplying. The side effects occur mainly because they also target some of the normal cells. Although we still use chemotherapy for some people with lung cancer, several new forms of treatment have become available in recent times. These new medications selectively target the cancer cells and generally cause fewer side effects compared to chemotherapy. The cancer doctor will explain this further.'

- Further tests will be done if he prefers to receive treatment.

  'If the decision is taken to try one of the new treatments, the cancer doctor will probably ask for further blood tests or suggest taking a small sample from the tumour in the lung. This will be done by a lung specialist, who will pass a long thin tube via the throat into the lung to get the sample. The results of these tests will help the cancer doctor choose a treatment that is likely to work best for him.'

- If he prefers to not receive treatment, the oncologist will recommend palliative measures to make sure he does not suffer.

  'If he prefers to not receive any treatment for the cancer, it does not mean that we won't do anything. We can still give him the treatments to manage his symptoms and make sure he does not suffer. In due course, I am sure the cancer doctor will refer him to the palliative team, who are experts on providing care towards the end of life. Let's discuss with your father to find out what his wishes are.'

She says she is willing to consider the treatment options but asks you not to tell her father about his diagnosis of cancer. She wants you to tell him that the fluid collection was due to infection.

In several parts of the world, including India, China, Japan, South-East Asia, and Middle East, families have a major influence in treatment decisions, especially for the elderly. It is also common for elderly people to ask doctors to 'have a discussion with their children'. Unlike in the Western world, family values usually take precedence over individual rights in these countries. Thus, with increasing migration and with societies becoming multi-cultural, these challenges are likely to be faced by doctors working in Western countries too.

Some families may go a step further and ask you not to disclose a terminal diagnosis to the patient, to spare them the mental distress during the final days. The argument against withholding the diagnosis is that the patient has the right to know (autonomy). It will be difficult to treat him without his consent. If he is not well informed, he is less likely to be compliant. If he finds out at a later date about his diagnosis from other sources, it is likely to affect the doctor–patient relationship. Hence, withholding information is probably justified only if the disclosure is likely to cause harm to the patient (e.g. the patient is likely to entertain suicidal thoughts) or in an emergency, when the patient is incapacitated.

- *Ask why she does not want you to reveal the diagnosis to her father.*

She tells you that she does not want him to get upset or distressed. She can't imagine how he would feel if he knew that the cancer was incurable and there was no guarantee that the treatments will keep things under control.

Tell her that:

- *Withholding the diagnosis from him could be counterproductive.*

   'I appreciate your concerns. However, if he asks us directly, we cannot lie. Even if he doesn't ask, I would suggest that we tell him the truth. If he finds out about his diagnosis through someone else at a later date, he will feel betrayed and lose his trust in the medical team. It'll affect his relationship with the medical team, and he might even stop following our advice. It is also difficult for you and your family to keep this away from him for a long time. If he is taken to a cancer clinic, for example, he will surely meet other patients with cancer there and start to guess that he, too, might have the same problem. I feel that it'll make him more distressed than how he would feel if we told him now.'

- *We need his consent to perform the biopsy or start him on treatment.*

   'We need his consent to obtain the sample from the lung or give him the treatments for the cancer. Without knowing the diagnosis, he won't be able to understand the benefits or risks of the proposed treatments. It is better to tell him, so that he knows what to expect.'

- *You will take care to break the news in a graded manner.*

   'We'll gently break the news in a graded manner. You and your family members can be present when we tell him. We'll start by asking how much he wants to know before talking to him. Once we tell him, I am sure it'll make you less anxious and enable you and your family members to work together with him. Contrary to what you think, he might actually take it well. It'll also help him plan better for the future and give him a dignified death.'

End the conversation by summarising the main points. Tell her that you would like to gently break the news to her father at the right time in her presence. Ask her to think about the reasons you mentioned for disclosing to him. If he prefers to receive treatment, the oncologist will discuss the next steps. Tell her that she can get in touch with you if she has any questions in the interim.

SUMMARY

This scenario tests your skills in communicating with a daughter who wishes to keep the diagnosis of cancer away from her father. You will be expected to:

- Gently break the news about the diagnosis of advanced lung cancer to the daughter.
- Tell her that the cancer is incurable and the intent of treatment is to prolong life and control his symptoms.
- Briefly discuss the treatments for lung cancer.
- Explain why you would discourage withholding the diagnosis from her father.
- Reassure her that you can gently break the news to him in a graded manner in the presence of family members.

You should balance his right to know (autonomy) against her concern that he will become mentally distressed if the bad news is broken (non-maleficence).

The 37-Year-Old Man with Gonorrhoea Who Asks You Not to Tell His Wife about His Diagnosis

This 37-year-old man was admitted two days ago with a three-day history of fever, joint pains, and skin rash. He described the joint pains as migratory, mainly involving the hands, knuckles, knees, and ankles. Skin rash was present over the forearms. Systems enquiry was entirely unremarkable.

His past medical history is blameless, and he does not take any regular medication. He drinks one or two glasses of wine during weekends but does not smoke or use recreational drugs. He works as an interior designer and lives with his wife and three young children.

Of note, he recently went on a short holiday to Thailand with two of his school friends and returned home three days prior to the onset of his illness. He denied having sexual intercourse with anyone other than with his wife.

His temperature on admission was 37.5°C, but the rest of the vital parameters were satisfactory. There were no signs of synovitis or tenosynovitis on examination. There were a few pustular-looking rashes over the volar aspect of his distal upper limbs. The rest of the examination was unremarkable. His laboratory tests showed elevated total white cell count with neutrophilia. His liver function tests, renal function, and urinalysis were normal. C-reactive protein was elevated. He was empirically commenced on intravenous ceftriaxone and given regular diclofenac.

Blood cultures drawn at the time of admission have just been reported as showing Gram-negative diplococci in pairs, identified as *Neisseria gonorrhoeae*. Your task is to discuss the results of the blood culture and the next steps with him. You are the medical registrar on the ward. You have not met him before, as he was transferred to your ward from the acute medical unit only this morning.

His clinical presentation is in keeping with disseminated gonococcal infection (DGI). *Neisseria gonorrhoeae* infection causes urethritis, which may manifest as painful urination or urethral discharge. However, a majority of patients, especially women, may be asymptomatic. In DGI, the organism invades the bloodstream and spreads to distant sites in the body. Clinical features of the most common type of DGI, also known as arthritis-dermatitis syndrome, include fever, malaise, migratory polyarthralgia, tenosynovitis, and pustular or petechial skin rash. Less commonly, DGI presents with septic gonococcal arthritis. Rare complications include meningitis, endocarditis, and osteomyelitis.

To make a diagnosis, specimens should be collected from mucosal sites (e.g. urethra, vagina, endocervix, pharynx, rectum) and sent for culture and polymerase chain reaction. In DGI, blood and synovial fluid samples should be sent for culture. However, the blood culture may be positive in only about 50% of the patients with DGI, as the bacteraemia is not continuous. The antibiotic of choice for the treatment of gonorrhoea is ceftriaxone (single dose for uncomplicated infection and a seven-day course for DGI).

- Introduce yourself, and confirm his identity. Tell him that you have come to discuss his blood test results. Ask how he is and what he has been told already.

He says his joints feel better with the anti-inflammatory pills. He hasn't been told much except that he may have an infection in his blood.

Tell him that:

- *His blood culture result is positive for gonococcus.*

  '*I am glad to hear that the anti-inflammatory pills are helping. [Pause.] The blood test results have confirmed our suspicions. We found a bug called gonococcus in your blood. This explains your fever, tiredness, joint pains, and the blisters on your skin. The antibiotic that we are giving you should help treat this infection.*'

- *Gonococcal infection is sexually transmitted.*

  '*I must tell you something, which may be a bit embarrassing. [Pause.] Gonococcus is an infection that is transmitted from one person to another by sexual intercourse.*'

He seems taken aback but does not say anything.

- *You should now obtain a detailed sexual history.* Start with:

  '*I hope you won't mind if I ask you some sensitive questions. I know you told the other doctor that you didn't have sexual intercourse with anyone other than your wife, but I would like to go over the details once again.*'

After some initial reluctance, he sheepishly admits that he visited a commercial sex worker in Thailand.

- Ask further questions about his sexual exposure.

Was it a man or woman? Did he use a condom? Has he had any genitourinary symptoms, like urethral discharge or painful urination, since the exposure? Has he had previous encounters with commercial sex workers? Has he been tested for HIV in the past? When was the last time he had intercourse with his wife? Was it protected or unprotected? Is the wife well?

He says the sex worker was a young woman. The condom slipped and fell when he had intercourse with her. He has not had any discharge from his penis or pain on passing urine. That was the first time he visited a commercial sex worker. He has never been tested for HIV. He had unprotected intercourse with his wife a day after he came back from Thailand. She is well and has not reported any symptoms. He says it never occurred to him that he can catch an infection from the sex worker, and he is deeply remorseful for what he has done.

Tell him that:

- *You would like to screen him for other sexually transmitted infections.*

'I can see that you did not expect this. Whatever has happened has happened. Let's talk about what we should do from here on apart from treating your current infection. First, I would recommend testing for other infections that are transmitted by having sex. We'll take a blood and urine sample to test for those infections.'

- *You would encourage him to disclose this to his wife so that she, too, can be tested.*

'I know it's not easy, but I would strongly encourage you to tell your wife, so that she, too, can be tested. As you had intercourse with her after coming back from Thailand, it is possible that you have passed the infection to her.'

He gets very distressed when you tell him that he must disclose this matter to his wife. 'No way! I can never do that', he says. He asks why he must tell her when she has no symptoms.

- *Explain why you are asking him to tell the wife.*

'I can totally understand, but please allow me to explain why I'm asking you to do that. First of all, just because she is well and has no symptoms does not mean that she hasn't caught the infection from you. Most women with gonococcal infection do not experience any symptoms. Second, if she is tested and found to have the infection, we can give her the necessary treatments. Third, and most important, I am concerned that if she is not treated, she could potentially develop some complications. The infection can cause inflammation of the womb and the ovaries, leading to long-standing pain and suffering. There is also a small chance for the infection to spread throughout the body and make her quite unwell. It could turn serious if it affects the layers around the brain, the heart, or the bones. Please think about it.'

- *Tell him if she gets symptoms and seeks medical advice, she will find out from the doctor.*

'If she develops symptoms and seeks medical advice, she'll find out from the doctor, and it'll only make things more difficult for you. I must also tell you that if you are treated and she is not, you can once again get the infection back from her if you continue to have unprotected intercourse with her, because you don't develop immunity against gonococcus. If you suddenly abstain from sex or start using a condom, she'll wonder why you are doing that, and it'll only make things more complicated.'

- Tell him that *you would also recommend an HIV test.*

'I realise that all this is too overwhelming for you, but I would also strongly recommend doing an HIV test. It's the virus that causes AIDS. If your result is negative, we must repeat *the test again after three months. If your result is positive either now or later, we should then test your wife as well. It's important because there are very effective treatments for HIV. Without treatment, HIV could become serious and shorten the lifespan.'*

He says you can do whatever test you want on him but he is still not sure how he can tell his wife. He then asks if you will support him if he tells her in your presence that he got the infection by using a public toilet. He also asks if you will prescribe the antibiotic for gonococcus and he will somehow make her take it.

- **Tell him that you cannot lie to his wife.**

'I'm afraid I cannot lie and won't be able to support you in this. In the United States, an antibiotic prescription for partners is handed to people with some sexually transmitted infections, but that's done only if the partners won't be able to come to the clinic to see a doctor. It's done with the good intention to treat them early. The prescription is given under the assumption that the partners will be told they could have caught the infection. It's never right to ask someone to take the antibiotics without telling why they must take them. Your wife deserves to receive the right treatment in the proper way.

'Moreover, if you are found to have other infections, she needs to be tested for those as well. Infections like gonococcus, as I said, could cause serious complications, and HIV will last a lifetime.'

'Expedited partner treatment', mostly practiced in the USA, is the practice of treating sexual partners of patients diagnosed with gonococcus or chlamydia without a prior medical examination. It is done only if the partner is unable to come to the clinic. The patient is given a prescription in the partner's name for a single dose of cefixime to treat gonococcus, and a seven-day course of doxycycline to treat chlamydia. Written information is handed to the patient to be passed to the partners so that they understand why they have been asked to take the antibiotics.

He asks if the information that he has shared with you will remain confidential. He says he is worried that you will call his wife and tell her if he doesn't.

- **Tell him that it is best for him to disclose to her.**

'It is best if she hears it from you than from any of us. If you prefer, I can ask a counsellor to guide you on how to gently break the news to her.

'To answer your question directly, yes, if someone is unable to break the news even after repeated requests and we feel that the partner is likely to suffer harm, I'm afraid we cannot then keep that information confidential anymore. We, however, do that as a last resort and only after very careful consideration of the risks to both parties. We'll never do that without telling you.'

End the conversation by telling him that you understand his difficulties but the wife deserves to know for the reasons you mentioned. Tell him that you will continue the antibiotics for the gonococcal infection, screen him for other sexually transmitted infections, and come back and talk to him later about the HIV test. Reassure him once more that you will never tell the wife without informing him.

The ethical dilemma for the clinician is the conflict between upholding confidentiality and the potential harm to the wife. The first step is to encourage him to tell his wife, although we can understand that it will be very difficult for him to openly tell her that he visited a sex worker and has possibly passed the infection to her.

Although we owe a duty of confidentiality, we owe a wider duty to protect the health of the public. If he refuses to tell the wife even after repeated requests, we may have to breach confidentiality and let her know *after* informing him. In such cases, it is always best to discuss with your peers and seek legal advice from the defence body. The General Medical Council in the UK states that 'if the patient refuses consent, disclosing confidential information may be justified in the public interest if failure to do so may expose others to a risk of death or serious harm'.

SUMMARY

This scenario tests your skills in convincing a husband to tell his wife, to whom he may have transmitted a sexually acquired infection. You will be expected to:

- Tell him that the blood culture has reported gonococcus.
- Obtain a sexual history.
- Discuss the treatment of disseminated gonococcal infection, and recommend screening for other sexually transmitted infections, including HIV.
- Tell him that his wife should be tested and treated.
- Encourage him to tell the wife, and clearly explain why.
- Make it clear that you cannot support his unethical suggestions.

You will not be expected to have convinced him, and it is indeed impossible to do that within ten minutes. However, you will get an unsatisfactory mark if you do not manage to clearly convey the importance of disclosing the matter to his wife or you promise to uphold the confidentiality.

A variation of this scenario is talking to a taxi driver who continues to drive his cab after being diagnosed with seizures. The same principles should be followed. He should be strongly encouraged to stop driving immediately (because of the danger to himself, his passengers, and others on the road) and inform the Driving Vehicles Licensing Authority (DVLA). You should gently tell him that if he fails to do that, you will have to let the DVLA know after informing him.

Challenging Patients and Relatives

Case 23

The 26-Year-Old Man Who Is Asking to Be Tested for Huntington's Disease

This 26-year-old man has been given an appointment to see you in the general medicine clinic as he wants to be tested for Huntington's disease (HD).

He is asking for this test because his 53-year-old father, who lives abroad with his mother, was recently diagnosed with HD.

- After the initial introduction, ask how you can help.

He says his mother recently took his father to see a neurologist because he was getting increasingly forgetful. His movements were becoming clumsy, which made him fall on a couple of occasions at home. The neurologist arranged a brain scan and some blood tests and told him that he had Huntington's disease. He also told him that his close family members were at higher risk of getting this condition and there was a blood test that can help predict this. He asks if you can arrange that blood test for him.

Huntington's disease (HD) is a neurodegenerative disorder that is inherited in an autosomal dominant manner. It is characterised by (1) movement disorders (unsteadiness of gait, choreiform movements, dystonia, bradykinesia, problems with speech and swallowing, eventually leading to a bedridden state), (2) cognitive impairment, and (3) psychiatric disturbance (depression, suicidal ideation, changes in personality and behaviour). Some describe HD as a combination of Alzheimer's dementia, Parkinson's disease, and amyotrophic lateral sclerosis. It is incurable.

HD is caused by CAG (cytosine, adenine, and guanine) trinucleotide repeat expansion in the gene that codes for huntingtin protein. Normal individuals have ≤26 CAG repeats in the huntingtin gene, but those with HD typically have ≥40 CAG repeats. Those with 27–35 CAG repeats are not at risk of developing HD (intermediate), while those with 36–39 CAG repeats may or may not develop symptoms (reduced penetrance). However, future generations of those with 27–39 repeats are at risk of developing HD because of subsequent expansion of CAG repeats. The age of onset of symptoms depends on the number of repeats. The higher the number of repeats, the earlier the onset of symptoms.

- Tell him that you are sorry to hear about his father, and *ask what he knows about HD*.

DOI: 10.1201/9781003533337-27

He says he does not know much about Huntington's disease except that it is a disease that affects the brain. He was scared to check online. He asks if you can explain what it is.

- *Explain HD in layman's terms* (speak slowly).

   'Huntington's disease is caused by a faulty gene. The faulty gene makes a protein that damages the cells in some parts of the brain. It leads to a gradual decline in mental functions, like thinking and memory. It causes uncontrolled movements of the body and makes the person clumsy and unsteady. The condition gradually gets worse over time. Eventually, the person loses the ability to walk, speak, or swallow and becomes bedridden and dependent on others.'

Note: It is good to give him a true picture of the general course of the disease so that he can make an informed decision about whether or not to have the test.

He says he is deeply upset to hear this. He asks if there is any treatment for this condition.

- Tell him that *there is no cure*.

   'At present, I am afraid there is no cure. There is also no treatment at present that can stop further progression or slow down the disease. However, there are medications that can suppress the uncontrolled movements and improve the mood. There is also a lot that we can do to support the needs of the person, like nursing care or assisting with mobility, feeding, and communication.'

He asks what his chances are of developing this condition.

- Tell him that before you answer that question, you would like to *find out more about him and his family members*.

Obtain a brief history. Has he been experiencing any of the symptoms that his father has? Does he have any medical problems? What is his occupation? Does he have any children? How many siblings does he have? How many siblings does his father have? Are they all well?

He says he feels well. He has none of the symptoms that his father is experiencing. He has no known medical problems. He is an investment banker. He is married and has a 2-year-old son. He and his wife are now trying for another baby. He is the eldest child in his family. He has a brother and a sister. His father has two older sisters, and they each have a daughter. As far as he is aware, no one else in his family has developed the symptoms of Huntington's disease.

- Tell him that *he and each of his two siblings have a one in two chance of developing the condition*.

   'Huntington's disease is passed from the affected parent to the children, as it is caused by a faulty gene. We have thousands of genes in our cells. All our genes have two copies. One comes from the father, and one from the mother.
   'A person with Huntington's disease has one normal copy and one faulty copy of a particular gene. You would have either got the normal or the faulty copy of that gene from your father. We don't know which one you got. If you have the normal copy, you

won't get the disease. If you have the faulty copy, you will get Huntington's disease in the future. So there is a one in two chance that you have inherited the faulty gene. Each of your siblings, too, has the same risk.'

- **Ask why he wants to have the blood test** to find out if he has the huntingtin gene.

He says he came to see you only because he learnt that close family members are at risk of getting the condition. Now that you have explained in detail, he is convinced that he wants the blood test. It will give him a huge sense of relief if the result shows that he hasn't got the faulty gene.

Tell him that:

- **You will refer him to a genetic counsellor.**

'I'll refer you to a genetic counsellor. A genetic counsellor educates people about genetic diseases and the implications of having genetic tests. The counsellor will explain the pros and cons of having the blood test. This is important because you must be mentally well prepared when the test result is out.

'If the result is positive, you'll have to live with the mental distress that you are going to get the disease long before you even get it. It may change your general outlook on life. On the positive side, knowing that you have the gene can help you plan for the future and live your life to the fullest until you get it. There are people who say they do not see the benefit in getting tested, as there is no treatment for the condition. They don't mind living with the uncertainty. The decision to get tested is entirely personal, and there is no right or wrong answer.'

He asks if this means that there is a 50% chance that his child has got it. He would also like to get his child tested if that is the case.

Tell him that:

- It depends on whether he has got it in the first place. Even if he has inherited the faulty gene, **the child cannot be tested until he is 18 years old.**

'Unless you have the faulty copy of the gene, your child is not at risk of developing Huntington's disease. If you do, there is a one in two chance that your child has got it. The risk is the same for your future children too. If you got the normal copy from your father, you are not at risk, and you will therefore not pass it to any of your children. But even if you are found to have the faulty gene, we cannot test your son until he is 18. We don't test children because they won't be able to understand the implications of a positive result.'

Note: Children below 18 years of age can be tested only if they exhibit symptoms of juvenile-onset HD in the opinion of a neurologist.

- **Pre-implantation genetic testing is possible** for future children.

'If you are found to have the faulty copy of the gene and wish to have more children, we can test the embryo before it is implanted into your wife's womb. We can collect your

sperms and fertilise your wife's eggs outside the body – we call this in vitro fertilisation, or IVF for short. It is possible to test the embryos for the faulty gene and implant one with the normal copy of the gene. If your wife is already pregnant, it is possible to do the tests with the fluid that circulates around the baby. You may then decide to abort the pregnancy if the baby is found to have the faulty gene.'

Note: For women who are already pregnant, testing the foetus with chorionic villus biopsy or amniocentesis is possible.

He says it is unlikely that he would try for another baby if he is found to have the faulty gene, but he will discuss it further with the genetic counsellor. He asks at what age he can expect to develop symptoms if he has inherited the faulty copy and if the disease will reduce the lifespan.

- Tell him that *the age of onset depends on the number of CAG repeats*.

  'It is hard to say precisely. Our genes have tiny units that are denoted by the letters C, A, and G. These three units keep repeating along the gene – in normal people, they repeat fewer than 26 times, but in those with Huntington's disease, they repeat at least 40 times or more. The age at which the symptoms begin depends on the number of times the three units repeat. People with a higher number of repeats tend to get it earlier. Most people tend to first notice the symptoms during their 30s or 40s.'

- *The disease reduces the lifespan.*

  'People with the condition usually die about 15–20 years after developing the first symptoms.'

End the discussion by telling him that you will refer him to a genetic counsellor and he can have the blood test only after that. If he has any further questions, he can ask the counsellor. Finish on a positive note and tell him, *'Research is very active in this field, so let's be optimistic and hope that some groundbreaking treatment will be discovered in the not-too-distant future'*.

There isn't enough time to discuss all the issues in ten minutes, but the relative may ask about the implications of a positive test result on obtaining life insurance.

- If the person has already got life insurance, the result of a subsequent predictive genetic test should not affect the premium.
- If the person hasn't got life insurance yet but intends to get one, he will be expected to disclose his father's diagnosis on the application. It is then up to the individual insurance company, which may decline the application or charge a higher premium.
- In the UK (the rules may be different in other countries), the insurance company cannot compel a person to have the predictive genetic test or, if the person has already had the test, ask for the result (unless the person is seeking to obtain more than £500,000 of life insurance).
- If the result of the predictive genetic test is negative, the person may wish to disclose the result, as he would be able to cut down the premium to the standard rate.

SUMMARY

This scenario tests your skills in communicating the pros and cons of having a predictive genetic test. You will be expected to:

- Find out what he already knows about HD and why he wants to have the blood test.
- Explain HD is layman's terms.
- Tell him that there is no cure.
- Tell him that there is a one in two chance that he has inherited the condition.
- He can be tested only after he has been counselled by a genetic counsellor because of the implications of a positive or negative result.
- Even if he is found to carry the huntingtin gene, his child cannot be tested until he turns 18. Pre-implantation diagnosis is, however, possible for his future children.

A variation of this case is talking to a woman whose sister was recently found to be BRCA (breast cancer gene) positive after being diagnosed with triple-negative breast cancer at an early age. You will be expected to:

- Find out about her sister's diagnosis of breast cancer.
- Ask if she herself has experienced any symptoms or been screened for cancer.
- Explain what BRCA gene is.

    'BRCA is a gene that reduces our risk of developing certain cancers. People who have a faulty BRCA gene are therefore at higher risk of developing certain cancers than the rest of the population. The cancer tends to occur in the breast or ovary in most women.'

- Tell her that there is a one in two chance that she has got the harmful variant of BRCA.
- Tell her that you will refer her to a genetic counsellor.
- Tell her about the implications of a positive or negative result. A positive result means that she is at increased risk of certain cancers (e.g. breast, ovarian, peritoneal in women, and breast and prostate in men). The cancer is likely to occur at an earlier age compared to the rest of the population. There is a small chance that she may never develop cancer. If the result is negative, her risk of cancer will be the same as the rest of the population.

- Briefly discuss the measures to reduce the risk of cancer, which may include (1) enhanced screening (starting at an earlier age and done more often), (2) preventive surgery (e.g. bilateral mastectomy with breast reconstructive surgery, bilateral salpingo-oophorectomy), or (3) chemoprevention (PARP inhibitors, tamoxifen, raloxifene).
- Discuss the risks to her current or future children.
- Tell her that her children need not be tested before they reach adulthood (usually deferred until the age of 25 in women and 35 in men, as cancer screening will not begin before that age even if the result is positive).

The 46-Year-Old Man Who Is Not Compliant with His Anti-Hypertensive Medication

> This 46-year-old man was diagnosed with hypertension about three months ago and commenced on ramipril. Prior to that, he was in good health. His fasting blood glucose, HbA₁c, lipids, renal function, and electrolytes were all found to be normal at that time.
>
> When he came for his blood test appointment this morning, the nurse found that his blood pressure was 164/100 mmHg. The reading was similar when it was repeated after some time.
>
> She has asked if you could advise him on the next steps to control his blood pressure. You are the registrar in the medical clinic.

- After the initial introduction, tell him about the purpose of the consultation. ('*The nurse who saw you earlier wanted me to have a word with you to see how we could improve your blood pressure.*'). Ask if he is well.

He says he feels fine but came to see you only because the nurse told him that his blood pressure was high. He asks what an ideal blood pressure reading is and what those numbers mean.

- Tell him that *his blood pressure reading is indeed high*.

  '*We aim for a blood pressure reading below 130/80. The top number denotes the pressure in the blood vessels when the heart is beating and pushing blood around the body. The bottom number is the pressure when the heart is relaxing between two beats. Your readings just now were around 160/100, which is quite high.*'

- *Ask if he takes ramipril every day* as advised (the most important question to ask).

He says was advised to take the blood pressure pill every day but he only takes it about once every three to four days.

Non-compliance to medication is a common problem. The usual reasons are (1) a lack of understanding of the intended purpose of the treatment (e.g. low literacy level, poor communication by the healthcare provider), (2) a lack of benefit, (3) side effects or fear of side effects, (4) forgetfulness or ignorance, (5) high drug costs, (6) a lack of symptoms (e.g. type

DOI: 10.1201/9781003533337-28

2 diabetes, hypertension, hyperlipidaemia, osteoporosis), or (7) a preference for alternative medicine. It is important to find out the reasons for non-compliance and to address them.

There are different types of non-compliance, such as (1) primary non-adherence (never initiated the drug), (2) non-persistence (stopped the drug after taking it for a certain period of time), and (3) non-conforming (e.g. skipping some doses, taking a lower or higher dose than what was prescribed). The problem may go unrecognised and result in serious health consequences. Some forms of non-compliance can also affect the community at large (e.g. spread of resistant mycobacteria due to non-compliance with anti-tuberculous treatment).

- *Ask why he does not take his ramipril regularly.* Also ask if he takes non-conventional or alternative medicine.

He says he has not experienced any symptoms from the high blood pressure, so there is no motivation for him to take the pill. Another reason is the irritating cough that he has had ever since he started taking the pill. He does not take any other form of treatment for his high blood pressure.

- Ask if he was forewarned about the cough before he was commenced on ramipril.
- Ask if he smokes or has other respiratory symptoms, like expectoration, haemoptysis, breathlessness, chest pain, fever, or weight loss.

He is unable to recall if he was told that the pill can cause cough. He has never had a cough like this before. It only started after he started taking this pill. He has never smoked. He denies expectoration, haemoptysis, breathlessness, chest pain, fever, or weight loss.

It appears that his non-compliance stems from (1) a lack of symptoms from the high blood pressure, (2) poor understanding of the intended benefits of treatment, and (3) side effects of the medication. These issues should be addressed one by one. Switching to an angiotensin receptor blocker (e.g. valsartan, losartan) should be recommended because of his cough, which is a well-known side effect of angiotensin-converting enzyme inhibitors.

Tell him that:

- *Hypertension often does not cause any symptoms.*

  'People with high blood pressure often do not experience any symptoms, so I am not surprised that you feel fine. The absence of symptoms does not mean, however, that the condition is harmless. It is important to take the pill every day, even if you don't feel unwell.'

- *Uncontrolled hypertension can lead to some complications.*

  'If the blood pressure is not controlled well and the reading remains persistently high for a long time, it can damage the lining of the blood vessels and increase your risk of a heart attack or stroke. Your heart must work harder to pump the blood against a higher pressure, so it can become weak in due course and make you get out of breath when you exert. There is also higher risk of the kidneys getting damaged. Diabetes and high blood pressure are, in fact, among the most common causes of kidney damage.'

'In some people, the blood pressure suddenly shoots up to a dangerously high level, causing swelling of the brain, bleeding in the brain, fluid collection in the lungs, or a sudden decline in kidney function. These problems, although not common, could be life-threatening.'

- **Keeping the blood pressure under control will reduce the risk of complications.**

'If we manage to keep the blood pressure under control, we can greatly reduce the chance of developing these complications. I am afraid there is no cure, which means we cannot take the problem away completely. You must continue taking the pills for life. Your blood pressure will remain under control as long as you take the pills. If you stop taking them, your blood pressure will rise again.'

What about the cough? he asks.

Tell him that:

- **Cough is a well-known side effect of ramipril.**

'We do see this problem in some people who take ramipril. You do not seem to have any other symptom to suggest that your cough is caused by a lung problem, so let's stop the ramipril. Your cough should go away once you stop it. If it doesn't, I'll arrange a chest X-ray.'

- **You would recommend an alternative anti-hypertensive medication.**

'I'd recommend an alternative pill that works just like ramipril but without causing the cough. The new pill, which is called losartan, should be taken once daily.
'There are some side effects of this new pill that you must be aware of. It can cause the blood pressure to drop suddenly when you stand up and make you feel dizzy. I would therefore suggest that, for the first week or two, you take the pill at night, before you go to bed. It should pass after the first few days, and you can then take the pill at any time that suits you.
'Just like ramipril, the new pill can cause a sudden decline in the kidney function. This is usually a problem in older people with narrowing of the blood vessels that supply the kidney – it is unlikely in someone of your age. It can also raise the potassium level in your blood. We'll regularly do blood tests to monitor your kidneys and potassium level if you take this pill.'

If he has no questions about losartan:

- Ask if he checks his blood pressure at home.

He says he doesn't check his blood pressure at home. He was advised to buy a blood pressure monitor, but he didn't want to waste money on it.

- Tell him that **you would recommend purchasing a home blood pressure monitor.**

'The blood pressure often goes up when people come to the clinic or hospital. It's usually a bit lower when they are at home. I would recommend buying a blood pressure monitor so that you can check your blood pressure at home, when you are more relaxed.

'You should select a monitor that goes around your upper arm, not the wrist or the fingers. It is possible to connect some monitors to your smartphone and transfer the readings to an app. It'll help us see your blood pressure readings on a graph and make adjustments to your treatment accordingly.'

He acknowledges your advice. He says he is happy to try losartan and consider buying a blood pressure monitor. He doesn't want to end up with a heart attack or stroke or to get any of the other complications that you mentioned.

- Ask him a few questions about his lifestyle so that you can provide some specific advice. Briefly ask about his exercise routine, dietary habits, alcohol consumption, sleep, and stress.

He says he is quite sedentary and doesn't exercise much. He admits that he eats out a lot and his dietary habits are not particularly healthy. He manages to sleep for about seven hours at night. He does not smoke but drinks a couple of large glasses of wine nearly every day. He is a human resources manager. His job is quite stressful. He lives with his wife and two teenage children.

Tell him that:

- In addition to taking the anti-hypertensive medication, *he should follow a healthy life-style to reduce his cardiovascular risk*.

'Taking the pills alone is not enough to reduce your future risk of heart attack or stroke. You should follow some healthy lifestyle habits as well. I would recommend going for a brisk walk most days of the week, but start gently and build slowly. I know it's not easy, but try to make some changes to your diet, like avoiding salty foods, cutting down fats and sugars, and consuming more veggies and fruits. You should perhaps cut down on the alcohol as well and look at ways of reducing your stress at work. Consider getting a pet dog – it'll reduce your stress and also help you go for a walk every day! You don't have to do all this at once. Take it one step at a time.'

End the conversation by summarising what you have agreed on. Tell him that you will pre-scribe losartan and it is important for him to take it regularly. His renal function and serum potassium should be measured soon after he starts losartan and at regular intervals thereaf-ter. In addition, he should follow the healthy lifestyle habits that you outlined. Tell him that the nurse will arrange a follow-up appointment.

SUMMARY

This scenario tests your skills in talking to a non-compliant patient with sub-optimally controlled hypertension. You will be expected to:

- Check his understanding of hypertension.
- Check his compliance with ramipril, and explore the reasons for his non-compliance.
- Address his lack of understanding about the absence of symptoms, and counsel him on the benefits of keeping the blood pressure under control.

- Suggest an alternative anti-hypertensive medication because of the side effect that he is experiencing with ramipril.
- Discuss the side effects of losartan and the precautions to be taken.
- Take the opportunity to emphasise the importance of healthy lifestyle measures to reduce his cardiovascular risk.

A variation of this case is talking to a patient with sub-optimally controlled rheumatoid arthritis who is not compliant with methotrexate for fear of side effects. You will be expected to:

- Explore her concerns.
- Explain to her that there is a higher risk of irreversible joint damage if the inflammation is not controlled adequately.
- Clarify the difference between symptom-relieving and disease-modifying treatments in rheumatoid arthritis.
- Tell her that methotrexate has been shown to suppress the underlying disease and limit joint damage.
- Reassure her that the benefits of methotrexate outweigh its risks, and talk about the measures that will help minimise the risk of side effects (e.g. folic acid to reduce the risk of stomatitis or bone marrow toxicity, regular blood tests to monitor her blood counts and liver function, limitation of alcohol intake, contraceptive precautions, pre-treatment checks like chest X-ray and hepatitis screen, pneumococcal vaccination).
- Discuss the alternative treatments (e.g. sulfasalazine) in case she has specific concerns with the use of methotrexate.

The 65-Year-Old Woman Who Wants to Try Herbal Treatment for Her Lymphoma

This 65-year-old woman was recently evaluated for prolonged fever, weight loss, tiredness, and cervical lymphadenopathy. After a meticulous workup that included lymph node and bone marrow biopsies, she was diagnosed with diffuse large B-cell non-Hodgkin's lymphoma.

The oncologist suggested combination chemotherapy when he saw her in the clinic two weeks ago. He told her that there is a high chance of remission with treatment as her lymphoma was in the early stage, but she asked for some time to decide if she wanted to go ahead with his suggestion.

She has now come to the oncology clinic for her follow-up appointment. The consultant has asked you to first see her and discuss with him later. You are the registrar in the clinic. The nurse who checked her vitals tells you that the patient expressed to her that she is not keen to receive chemotherapy and would prefer to try herbal treatments instead.

- After the initial introduction, tell her that the consultant is seeing patients in another room and you will discuss with him once you have seen her. Start by asking her how she is.

She tells you that she still feels quite unwell. When she came to see the consultant two weeks ago, he told her that the biopsy showed lymphoma. Although it wasn't pleasant news, she was relieved to finally get a diagnosis. He suggested a combination of injections and tablets to treat the lymphoma and told her that there was a very high chance of success with this approach. However, he mentioned a lot of side effects, which seemed quite dreadful.

She asks if she must really take such strong medicines and put up with all those side effects. She would rather try herbal treatments or something natural, as they are free of side effects.

- Tell her that you are sorry to hear that she feels quite unwell, and *ask what she understands about lymphoma*.

She says she knows that lymphoma is the cancer of the lymph glands. The consultant told her that the white blood cells in the lymph glands are multiplying without any control.

- *Ask if there are any side effects of chemotherapy that she is particularly concerned about.*
- *Ask why she wants to try herbal treatment* in particular.

How did she hear about it? Does she know anyone who has tried it, or has she consulted an alternative medicine practitioner?

She says she doesn't want to put harmful chemicals into her body. Her nephew died of a severe allergic reaction to an antibiotic many years ago, and she has generally been averse to taking medications since then. If her condition is not too bad, she would rather avoid taking Western medicine or anything that is artificial. She doesn't want to lose hair, become sick, or keep getting infections. She has always favoured natural treatments and has been reading up about herbal treatments on the internet. She has not seen any other practitioner and does not know anyone who has tried them.

Although a majority of patients with cancer use complementary and alternative medicine (CAM), more than half of them do not tell their treating physician about it, for fear of disapproval or because they perceive the treatment as safe and natural. *Complementary* treatments refer to those that are used *along with* conventional treatments, while *alternative* treatments are those that are used *in place of* conventional treatments.

You should use the time to (1) help her understand the diagnosis and its prognosis with and without treatment (her response indicates that she may not have fully grasped the seriousness of the condition), (2) explain the benefits and risks of the proposed conventional treatment, and (3) discuss the role of complementary and alternative treatments without being close-minded, dismissive, or judgemental so that she can make an informed choice. It is not necessary to have a thorough knowledge of CAM to have this discussion.

After expressing your sadness for the death of her nephew, tell her that:

- *Her lymphoma is in the early stage, and it is likely to spread if treatment is delayed.*

  'My consultant must have told you that your cancer is still in the early stages. He feels that there is a very high chance of success with the treatment that he is proposing. There is even a good chance of cure, which means the cancer will go away with treatment and it won't come back again. If the cancer goes away, we can stop the treatment after some time.

  'If we do not treat the cancer while it is still in the early stages, it could spread throughout the body pretty quickly and become life-threatening. Once the cancer becomes advanced, it'll become difficult to treat. The prospect of cure will gradually diminish as the cancer advances.'

- *Conventional treatments are indeed associated with some side effects.*

  'The treatment recommended by the consultant – we call this chemotherapy – stops the cancer cells from multiplying. Unfortunately, chemotherapy medicines also target some of the normal, fast-growing cells, like those in the hair root; the bowel lining; the inner part of the bone, where blood cells are produced; and the gonads, where sperms and eggs *are produced. This is the reason for the side effects, like hair loss, sickness, diarrhoea, and infertility. There is a higher chance of catching an infection because of the reduced production of white blood cells. Some of those medications can also cause an allergic reaction.'*

- **The team will take appropriate steps to minimise the side effects** as much as possible.

'We always take the necessary steps to minimise these side effects. You will be given other medicines along with chemotherapy to stop the sickness, prevent an allergic reaction, and increase the production of blood cells to reduce the risk of infection. We'll be doing regular blood tests so that we can start you on appropriate treatments as soon as the blood counts start falling. The hair loss is temporary. It'll grow back once you complete the treatment.'

Pause for a while, and invite any questions. Check her understanding of what you told her, particularly that the cancer is likely to advance without treatment.

If she has no questions, *discuss the pros and cons of the herbal treatments that she wishes to try*. First, convey to her that:

- You appreciate her willingness towards self-care.

'I applaud you for taking the effort to manage your own health.'

- Many people with cancer do try CAM treatments.

'Many people with cancer do try other forms of treatments in the hope that they will make them better without causing side effects. You are not alone.'

- You are not trained in CAM practices but will try to offer a balanced opinion so that she can make an informed choice.

'I'm afraid I only have limited knowledge of herbal treatments, as we do not receive formal training in the other forms of medicine, but I will try to tell you whatever I know.'

It is important to show appreciation, reassure her that she is not alone, and admit your own lack of authority on the subject. It will help convey open-mindedness, empathy, and humility and give her the impression that she can freely discuss her wishes and preferences with you.

Further tell her that:

- **CAM treatments may improve the symptoms but not treat the cancer.**

'In general, herbal or other forms of alternative medicine do not treat the cancer. They do not stop the multiplication of the cancer cells. I am therefore concerned that the cancer will continue to spread if you try those treatments on their own.

'Some herbal and natural treatments can, however, help the symptoms of cancer, like pain, sickness, tiredness, lack of energy, and low mood. They can improve your well-being

and make you feel better. You may be able to take them along with the medicines that we give you.'

- **Not all CAM treatments are safe.**

'Herbal treatments can also cause side effects. Natural does not mean that they are safe. Some herbal treatments may not be appropriate to use along with the chemotherapy medicines that we give you as they increase the risk of side effects or make the treatment less effective. There are many different types of herbal or natural treatments – we will let you know which ones are suitable for you to take.'

- **Many CAM practices or treatments are not evidence-based.**

'The chemotherapy medicines that we use undergo extensive testing in research studies. Approval is granted for the use of these medicines only if they are shown to work and the benefits outweigh the risks.

'We cannot say the same about alternative forms of medicine. There are so many different types, and not all of them undergo such rigorous testing. Natural supplements and herbs are not regulated in the same way that chemotherapy medicines are. There is so much that we do not know about many of those forms of treatment, so you should be cautious.'

End the discussion by summarising the main points. Tell her that now that she has heard about the pros and cons of both forms of treatment, she can make an informed choice and you will respect her wishes. She can take some more time to decide, but you hope that she will come to a decision soon, as the cancer can spread very quickly. Emphasise once again that alternative treatments can help treat the symptoms, but not the cancer. If she remains resistant to your suggestions, tell her that if a trial of alternative treatment fails, she can come back to discuss conventional treatment at any time.

SUMMARY

This scenario tests your skills on negotiating a plan with a patient who wishes to try alternative treatment for a potentially serious condition. You will be expected to:

- Find out what she understands about lymphoma and the treatment that was suggested by the consultant.
- Explore her reasons for wanting to try herbal treatment.
- Explain the benefits and risks of chemotherapy, and stress upon her that the lymphoma is likely to advance without treatment.
- Outline the precautions that will be taken to minimise the side effects of chemotherapy.
- When discussing CAM, (1) appreciate her willingness towards self-care, (2) reassure her that she is not alone, and (3) admit your own lack of authority on the subject.

- Explain to her that (1) CAM treatments may relieve some of the symptoms but not treat the cancer, (2) not all of them are safe, and (3) they are not regulated in the same way as conventional treatments are.
- If she remains resistant to your suggestions, tell her that you will respect her wishes and she can change her mind anytime.

Case 26

The 24-Year-Old Man with Difficult Asthma

This 24-year-old man was admitted to the acute medical unit (AMU) yesterday with an acute exacerbation of his asthma. He had presented with acute shortness of breath, wheezing, and cough.

He had asthma as a child and grew out of it, but his symptoms returned about two years ago. Spirometry at that time confirmed reversible airway obstruction. He was prescribed inhaled corticosteroid and long-acting beta agonist (fluticasone-salmeterol) twice daily.

However, in the last one year, he has visited the emergency department (ED) at least half a dozen times with acute exacerbation of his asthma. During each of his previous visits, he was managed in the ED with nebulised bronchodilators and sent home on a short course of oral corticosteroid. Of late, he had been using the reliever inhaler (salbutamol) about two to three times a week during the daytime and sometimes at night. His activities were not limited because of his asthma.

At the time of admission yesterday, he was unable to speak in full sentences. His vital signs revealed normal temperature, heart rate 104/minute, respiratory rate 28/minute, oxygen saturation 96% on room air, and blood pressure 116/76 mmHg. Widespread polyphonic rhonchi were heard on both sides. His full blood count and renal function were normal. A chest X-ray was not done. He was treated with nebulised bronchodilators and intravenous hydrocortisone.

His symptoms have markedly improved in the last 24 hours. His vital signs are back to normal. The plan is to switch to inhalers and discharge him later today, with advice to continue oral prednisolone for another three days. Your task is to talk to him about his frequent visits to the ED and suggest measures to improve his asthma control. You are the medical registrar in the AMU.

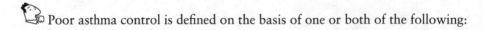 Poor asthma control is defined on the basis of one or both of the following:

1. Poor symptom control (frequent symptoms or use of the reliever inhaler more than twice a week, night-time awakening due to asthma, *or* limitation of activity by symptoms)
2. More than two exacerbations per year requiring oral corticosteroid for more than three days *or* more than one serious exacerbation per year requiring hospitalisation

134

DOI: 10.1201/9781003533337-30

In patients with difficult asthma, it is always useful to first ask yourself if the diagnosis is correct. There are several conditions that can mimic asthma, like chronic obstructive pulmonary disease, bronchiectasis, sarcoidosis, hypersensitivity pneumonitis, and heart failure. In this patient, it appears that the diagnosis of asthma is correct based on his clinical presentation and the finding of reversible airway obstruction on spirometry. He is using his reliever inhaler about two to three times a week and waking up at night with breathlessness and wheezing, which suggest that his asthma control is poor.

If the diagnosis is correct and control of asthma is poor, there are four key questions to ask:

1. Is he compliant with the treatment?
2. How is his inhaler technique?
3. Are there any ongoing triggers, like dust, smoke, pets, drugs (e.g. β blockers, aspirin, non-steroidal anti-inflammatory drugs), or recurrent upper respiratory tract infection?
4. Are there any comorbidities that are likely to worsen his asthma control (e.g. gastro-oesophageal reflux disease, rhino-sinusitis, obesity, obstructive sleep apnoea) *or* associated conditions (e.g. eosinophilic granulomatosis with polyangiitis, allergic bronchopulmonary aspergillosis)?

Non-adherence to treatment, poor inhaler technique, and ongoing environmental triggers are the most common reasons for poor asthma control. If none of these factors are found, the patient can be diagnosed with severe asthma and referred to a respiratory physician for escalation of treatment (e.g. tiotropium, theophylline, montelukast), phenotyping, or biologic treatment (e.g. anti-IgE drug like omalizumab, anti-IL-5 drugs like mepolizumab and benralizumab).

- Introduce yourself, and confirm his identity. Tell him that you have come to talk to him about the control of his asthma. Ask how he is.
- *Check his understanding of asthma*, and ask what he feels about coming to the hospital so often with acute exacerbations.

He says he feels almost back to normal. He had asthma as a child. It went away when he was 12 or 13 but came back about two years ago. His GP made the diagnosis of asthma after arranging some breathing tests. She prescribed a purple inhaler to use twice daily and a blue inhaler to use whenever he felt breathless. She gave him a leaflet about asthma, but he only glanced at it briefly. He admits that he hasn't got a full grasp of the condition. His understanding of asthma is that the lungs become tight.

He says the blue inhaler usually helps. He uses it about two or three times a week and sometimes at night. He comes to the hospital only when the blue inhaler proves unhelpful or the attack is severe.

- *Explain asthma in layman's terms.*

  'We'll talk about how we can improve the control of your asthma. Before that, let me first explain what happens in asthma.

  'The air that we breathe passes through the airways in the lungs. During an asthma attack, the muscles around your airways become tight. The insides of your airways become swollen and produce more mucus. This narrows the space for the air to freely *move in and out of your lungs. It makes your breathing harder and produces the whistling noise.*

The airways become narrow when you are exposed to an external particle, like dust, smoke, pollen, virus, or a medication. In some people, exercise or cold weather can trigger an attack. The airways are normal at other times. This is the reason you get intermittent attacks of breathing trouble and feel normal at other times.'

- Tell him that you would like to **find more about him and his asthma**. Keep this brief.

Ask about his compliance to the preventive inhaler, inhaler technique, occupation, smoking habit and alcohol intake, pets at home, medications taken, allergies, comorbidities, family history, and vaccinations received.

He says he often forgets to use his purple inhaler, as he feels fine most of the time. The GP taught him how to use the inhaler. His work is office-based. He is not exposed to dust or other irritants in the workplace, but the flooring in his house is carpeted. He started smoking at the age of 18 and used to smoke about ten cigarettes a day. He cut it down to five cigarettes a day after he was diagnosed with asthma. He does not drink alcohol, as wine tends to trigger an attack of asthma.

He has a pet dog. He has had the dog for the last two years. He has no drug or food allergies. His symptoms are not triggered by exercise or cold weather. He does not take any oral medication. He does not suffer with stuffiness in his nose or acid reflux symptoms. He lives on his own but doesn't think he snores at night. There is no one in his family with asthma. He has not received any vaccines as an adult apart from the COVID-19 vaccines some years back.

There are several issues that need to be addressed, including his (1) non-compliance to the preventive inhaler, (2) inhaler technique, (3) smoking habit, (4) possible exposure to dander from his pet dog, and (5) vaccination record.

Tell him that:

- **It is important to be compliant with the preventive inhaler.**

    'An attack of asthma could be dangerous and life-threatening. The purple inhaler is supposed to prevent the attacks. It has two medicines in it. One is a steroid, which helps reduce the swelling in the airways, and the other is a medicine that helps relax the muscles around the airways and make them wider. The second medicine is similar to the blue inhaler, except that its effect will last about 12 hours. The purple inhaler should be used twice daily, even if you feel well.

    'Using the blue inhaler so often and frequently taking short courses of steroids are not the ideal way to manage your asthma. In the long run, repeated courses of steroids can cause some unwanted side effects, like weakness of the bones, rise in blood pressure, rise in blood sugar, and weight gain.'

- **You will refer him to an asthma nurse to check his inhaler technique.**

    'It is equally important to use the inhaler correctly; otherwise, you won't get enough medicine into your lungs. I'll ask our asthma nurse to see you before you go home, so that she can check your technique.'

- *Tobacco smoking is a common trigger for asthma.*

'I would strongly encourage you to stop smoking. I appreciate you for managing to cut down to five cigarettes a day, but it is important that you stop completely.

'Cigarette smoke can not only trigger the attacks of asthma but also increase the chance of damage to the lungs. Your GP will be able to prescribe nicotine replacement therapy if you are struggling to quit – it has nicotine in it, but without the other harmful chemicals. It'll help control your cravings while you are trying to quit.'

- *He may be reacting to his pet dog.*

'As I said earlier, your airways can become narrow when they are exposed to certain triggers. This is not easy for me to say, but I wonder whether you are reacting to your dog. People with asthma sometimes react to the skin cells that are shed by animals that have fur or feather.'

He interrupts you and says he will not follow your advice if you suggest that he must give away his dog. He shares a close bond with his dog, and he can't even think about it.

- *Provide advice on minimising exposure to his pet dog.*

'I understand. I was going to suggest a few things to minimise your exposure to the skin cells that your dog is shedding. It's important to clean your dog regularly, which I am sure you do, but if possible, please ask someone else to do it. If you must do it yourself, I'd suggest that you wear a dust mask. Pets often rub along the furniture and deposit their skin cells on the surface, so make sure your furniture is wiped regularly. It's a good idea to make your bedroom a pet-free zone and have an air cleaner at home. I hope these measures work and you don't have to give your dog away.

'It is possible to do tests to find out if you are allergic to your dog. I'll refer you to an allergy specialist, who can help with this.'

- *Provide advice on minimising exposure to other allergens.*

'You should find out what triggers your symptoms and try to avoid them. Avoid smoky environments and exposure to dust and pollen. Keep your windows closed during the pollen season, and make sure your pillows, mattresses, and bedding have covers. Remove all carpets and rugs, and replace them with wooden floors. Do not take anti-inflammatory tablets like ibuprofen, as they can trigger an attack.'

- Tell him that **you would recommend the flu and pneumococcal vaccines.**

'Viruses and other infections often trigger an attack of asthma. I'd recommend getting the flu shot every year to reduce the risk of getting the flu, and the pneumonia vaccine to protect you against some common bacteria that cause lung infection.'

End the discussion by summarising the main points and telling him what will happen next. Tell him that you will arrange to follow him in the clinic and consider specialist referral for escalation of therapy if the aforementioned measures prove unhelpful.

SUMMARY

This scenario tests your skills in exploring the reasons for poor asthma control in a young patient and addressing them. You will be expected to:

- Check his understanding of asthma and explore the reasons for his poor control.
- Address his non-compliance.
- Offer to check his inhaler technique.
- Advise him to stop smoking.
- Sensitively provide advice on minimising exposure to his pet dog.
- Offer some tips to minimise exposure to other allergens.

A variation of this scenario is talking to a young patient with recurrent diabetic ketoacidosis (DKA). You should (1) check her understanding of diabetes, (2) explain the seriousness of DKA, (3) explore the reasons for recurrent admissions with DKA and address them (e.g. non-compliance, incorrect injection technique, dietary indiscretion, substance abuse, psychological factors like depression, poor social circumstances), and (4) offer to seek specialist opinion and refer for diabetes education.

The 63-Year-Old Woman Whose Husband Asks You Not to Discharge Her

This 63-year-old woman with a background history of impaired glucose tolerance and hyperlipidaemia was admitted eight days ago with a six-month history of gradually worsening breathlessness and dry cough.

Her high-resolution computed tomography scan showed evidence of interstitial lung disease (ILD) with a combination of ground glass and fibrotic changes. The results of her lung function tests were in keeping with a restrictive pattern. Her echocardiogram showed an ejection fraction of 60% and normal pulmonary artery systolic pressure. The relevant autoantibody results were negative. She declined a lung biopsy. She was discussed in a multi-disciplinary meeting with the respiratory physician and radiologist, and their opinion was that her ILD was most likely idiopathic.

The respiratory consultant has commenced her on 40 mg of prednisolone per day (0.6 mg/kg) along with co-trimoxazole (for pneumocystis prophylaxis) and vitamin D. She was given influenza and pneumococcal conjugate vaccines (PCV-13). Long-term oxygen therapy was not considered yet, as her oxygen saturations were satisfactory. Her blood glucose rose soon after she started prednisolone, so she was commenced on subcutaneous insulin.

The respiratory consultant has arranged to see her in his clinic in a month to assess her response to steroid. The diabetic nurse has trained her to self-inject the insulin and monitor the capillary blood glucose at home. She has arranged to see her in the clinic on the same day when she comes to see the respiratory consultant. Your consultant told her during rounds this morning that she can be discharged home. However, her husband, who has just arrived on the ward, is unhappy to take her home. She has asked if you could talk to her husband. You are the medical registrar on the floor.

- After introducing yourself and confirming the identity of the husband, ask what he has been told already and find out what his concerns are.

The husband says they were told that her lungs were inflamed and scarred. He knows that the lung doctor has started her on steroid pills to improve her breathing. However, he doesn't think she is ready to be discharged because she is still breathless and her problem hasn't been sorted fully.

DOI: 10.1201/9781003533337-31

He is worried that he wouldn't know what to do if she became more breathless at home. Even if he decides to bring her to the hospital, he feels that the waiting time in the emergency department (ED) is horrendously long. It wasn't a pleasant experience when she was admitted this time, and he doesn't want to go through that again. He is also concerned that her blood sugar might go up further. He says the whole thing is too complex for a non-medical person like him to handle. He asks if you could send her home after her breathing becomes normal.

The husband seems to have some misconceptions, anxieties, and unrealistic expectations that need to be addressed. You should use the time to tell him (1) what you have done during her inpatient stay so far, (2) why further inpatient stay is not necessary, and (3) what post-discharge plans have been put in place to ensure safe discharge.

Tell him that:

- *Her breathlessness is due to ILD.*

'Yes, you're right. The scan and the breathing tests showed inflammation and scarring in her lungs. We do not know why she has developed this problem. There are some medical conditions that can cause inflammation of the lungs, but we did not find any evidence of those in her.'

- *She has been started on steroids for her ILD.*

'If her lung inflammation is not controlled well, it can lead to further scarring and damage. The lung doctor has therefore started her on steroid pills in the hope that they will control the inflammation and reduce further scar formation.

'At present, it is not clear how much of her breathing problem is due to ongoing inflammation and how much of it is due to damage that has already occurred. If her breathing trouble is mostly due to inflammation, it should improve with steroids. If her breathing trouble is mostly due to damage, the steroids may not help much.'

- *There is no cure for her lung problem.*

'I am afraid her breathing may never return to normal, as there is already some damage to the lungs that cannot be reversed. She will therefore continue to experience some breathing trouble when she exerts herself. We are hoping to improve her breathing with steroids, but as I said, it largely depends on how much of her breathing trouble is due to inflammation. If the inflammation does not respond well to the steroid, the lung doctor will discuss the next steps when he sees her in clinic.'

- *There is no need for her to stay in the hospital anymore.*

'It may take some weeks before we know if the steroid pills are helping to reduce the inflammation in the lungs. This is the reason the lung doctor has arranged to see her in his clinic in a month. There is no need to keep her in the hospital anymore, because there is nothing further for us to do until then.

'Staying in the hospital for too long will increase her risk of catching an infection – these infections are harder to treat than the ones that we catch outside the hospital. Staying in the hospital is only necessary for very ill patients or those who need treatments that cannot be given at home. I would suggest that you take her home and continue the steroid pills as per the advice of the lung doctor.'

The husband says he understands all that but asks you to put yourself in his shoes and think. He doesn't know what he should do if her breathing gets worse, other than bringing her back to the hospital.

- *Give him a realistic idea of her prognosis.* Tell him that her breathing may gradually worsen if the lung disease progresses and there is no response to steroid.

'*It is possible that her breathing will gradually continue to worsen, especially if she doesn't respond to the steroid pills. She should modify her activities depending on her abilities and avoid too much exertion. If the lung problem worsens to the extent that she is unable to get enough oxygen to her blood, the lung doctor may recommend giving oxygen continuously. He will then arrange for her to receive oxygen at home using a device called an oxygen concentrator.*

'*If, on the other hand, her breathing suddenly gets worse, I would suggest that you first check her oxygen level in the blood with the pulse oximeter – the probe that you place on the finger. If the reading is below 94%, please bring her to the hospital, because we should find out the reason for the sudden drop in her oxygen level. A lung infection is the usual cause for sudden worsening of the breathing.*'

- *You have taken some steps to reduce her risk of infection.*

'*Scarring in the lungs can increase her risk of infection. To reduce her risk of infection, we have given her the flu and pneumonia vaccines. We have started her on a pill called Bactrim, which she must take three times a week. This pill will reduce her risk of getting infected with an unusual bug called* Pneumocystis, *which mainly occurs in people who take a high dose of steroid.*'

He says he does not want to wait in the ED for several hours. He asks for your phone number so that he can first call you for advice before bringing her to the hospital.

Tell him that:

- *Patients are prioritised in the ED.*

'*I am sorry to hear that you did not have a pleasant experience in the ED this time. Let's hope the need does not arise, but please do not be discouraged from visiting the ED because of what happened this time. The waiting times can be up and down. The staff in the ED always try their best to prioritise the patients and attend to those who need more urgent attention first.*

'*I am sure that if she comes in with sudden worsening of her breathing, someone will attend to her promptly. If the problem does not warrant treatment in the hospital, the emergency doctor will provide advice and discharge her. Keeping her in the hospital for a longer time in anticipation that things will get worse in the future is not the right approach.*'

- *You will provide the contact details of the hospital.*

'*I only carry a personal phone, and we all work for only a certain number of hours. We keep moving between different teams. We sometimes go on leave. I can give you the contact details of our department – you can leave a message, and someone will get back to you during office hours.*

'If the problem needs urgent attention, please do not wait for us to get back to you. Bring her to the hospital right away or call the ambulance.'

What about the blood sugar? he asks. He says he is worried that her blood sugar will go up.

- Tell him that *she should follow the advice of the diabetic team.*

'The blood sugar control will hopefully improve when the lung doctor starts to taper the dose of the steroid. Until then, she should follow the advice of the diabetic nurse and inject insulin regularly. If she must continue taking steroids for a long time, the diabetic team may start her on tablets to control the blood sugar with or without the insulin. If the blood sugar reading is high and you are not sure what to do, you can leave a message with the diabetic nurse and she will call you back. As you know, she is going to see her on the same day when you come to see the lung doctor.'

End the discussion by summarising the main points and reiterating what he should do in case of an emergency. Tell him, *'Just because we are discharging her does not mean that we will stop caring for her and she is off our radar. It just means that we will continue to care for her in a different setting'.*

SUMMARY

This scenario tests your skills in talking to an anxious husband who does not wish to take his wife home until she gets well. You will be expected to:

- Find out what the husband has been told already, and explore his concerns.
- Explain the results of the investigations and the treatments given so far.
- Explain why there is no need to stay in the hospital anymore.
- Explain what post-discharge plans have been put in place to ensure safe discharge.
- Provide some guidance on what he should do if her breathing gets worse or the blood sugar reading is very high.
- Allay his anxieties regarding the long waiting times in the emergency department, and set some realistic expectations.

The 42-Year-Old Man with Non-Specific Back Pain Who Demands a Scan

This 42-year-old man presented to the emergency department (ED) earlier this morning with a three-day history of low back pain. He said the pain began suddenly, with no preceding trauma or unusual physical activity. It has since neither improved nor worsened.

The pain is localised to the back, and it does not radiate down his legs. There are no neurological symptoms in his legs like weakness or numbness, problems with urination or defecation, or systemic symptoms, like fever, sweats, or weight loss. His past medical history is blameless. In particular, there is no history of cancer or tuberculosis, and he has never suffered with back pain before. He has been taking ibuprofen and paracetamol three times a day, but they do not afford much relief. His father is known to have ankylosing spondylitis. His job is office-based. He hasn't been able to go to work for the last three days because of the pain.

The ED doctor diagnosed him with non-specific low back pain. She wanted to discharge him with some general advice and regular analgesia, but he is insisting on getting a scan of his back. She has asked if you could talk to him. You are the medical registrar.

- After introducing yourself, tell him that you are sorry to hear that he has been struggling with pain. Briefly ask about his back pain, and *find out why he thinks he needs a scan*.

He says his father has suffered with back pain since his late teens. He used to visit the GPs regularly, but they kept ignoring his pain for many years and attributed it to the nature of his job, which was manual. He was eventually diagnosed with ankylosing spondylitis at the age of 40 when he developed severe back pain one day. The X-rays showed ankylosing spondylitis and a fracture of the backbone at that time. He is keen to get a scan of his back because he is aware that ankylosing spondylitis runs in families. He says he doesn't want to find out that he has got this condition after breaking the backbone like his father.

He confirms that he developed back pain three days ago. He has never suffered with back pain before, and his back has never been stiff in the mornings. His joints are not painful or swollen. He has not been diagnosed with psoriasis, inflammatory bowel disease, or uveitis. His immediate family members (two sisters, son, and daughter) are all fine, with no musculoskeletal complaints.

DOI: 10.1201/9781003533337-32

It appears that he has developed some deep-rooted beliefs during his childhood because of the delayed diagnosis of ankylosing spondylitis in his father (e.g. '*Doctors can be wrong*', '*If I develop back pain, I should get a scan to find out if I have developed ankylosing spondylitis*', '*Ankylosing spondylitis is a serious condition, and it is important to diagnose it early*'). Any episode of back pain will trigger this chain of thoughts and force him to seek a medical opinion.

He does not seem to have any features of axial spondyloarthropathy or red flags to suggest other diagnoses, such as cancer, infection, vertebral compression fracture, or nerve root compression. His presentation is in keeping with non-specific low back pain, also known as simple back pain. Patients with simple back pain cannot (and should not) be provided with a precise anatomical or pathological diagnosis. The outlook is good, with a majority of patients improving within days to weeks. Poor understanding of the problem can lead to unhelpful thoughts, emotions, and behaviours ('yellow flags') and turn it into a chronic pain problem. It is therefore important to not only allay his anxieties about ankylosing spondylitis but also reassure him about the generally good outlook of simple back pain.

Tell him that:

- *His presentation is not in keeping with ankylosing spondylitis.*

    '*I am sorry to hear about your father. I hope he is well now. I do not feel that your back pain is due to ankylosing spondylitis. Ankylosing spondylitis, as you may have already gathered, is a condition that causes inflammation of the ligaments, the rope-like structures that connect the backbones together. In due course, the inflammation leads to hardening of the ligaments, which makes the back very stiff and restricts the movements.*
    '*Ankylosing spondylitis usually starts in the late teens or early 20s, not so late at the age of 42. The back pain begins insidiously, and it progresses very slowly over several months to years, whereas your pain came on more suddenly and it has only been there for the last three days. In ankylosing spondylitis, the back feels very stiff in the mornings for the first few hours and gradually eases as the day progresses, which is not what you are describing. Some people may also develop swollen joints or have associated skin, bowel, or eye inflammation, which you do not have. The risk of ankylosing spondylitis is indeed higher among family members, but it is not 100%.*'

Note: If you tell him in one line that his back pain is not due to ankylosing spondylitis, he will not be reassured. It is worth spending some time to clearly explain your reasoning.

- *His presentation is in keeping with simple back pain.*

    '*Your description is in keeping with what we call as simple back pain. It simply means that the pain is not due to an underlying medical condition. We do not exactly know what causes this kind of back pain. It may be due to tightness of the muscles in the back. It is a very common problem. Many of us will experience this kind of pain at some point in our life.*
    '*Although we do not know what causes simple back pain, we know that in a vast majority of people, the pain goes away within a few days to few weeks.*'

What is the harm in doing a scan just to make doubly sure? he asks.

- Tell him that *there is no benefit in doing a scan and it may be counterproductive.*

  '*We ask for a scan only if we suspect an underlying medical condition. You do not have any worrying features to suggest that your back pain is caused by an underlying medical condition, so there is no point in getting a scan. A scan may show some wear and tear changes in most people, but those changes will not explain your pain or change the treatment in any way. Occasionally, the finding of something incidental on the scan may lead to further unnecessary testing and cause needless anxiety.*

  '*We also know that people with simple back pain do not get better while they are waiting for the scan, which can take some time. This is because the thought that there is something wrong with the back can delay their recovery. I don't want you to feel that there is something wrong with your back and we need to find out what it is.*'

He says he only knows about ankylosing spondylitis. What other medical conditions can cause back pain, and what are those worrying features that you are referring to? he asks.

- *Reassure him that he does not have any red flags* suggestive of cancer, infection, fracture, and cord or nerve root compression.

  '*A small number of people with back pain may have an underlying problem, like cancer, infection, fracture of the backbone, or pressure on the spinal cord or nerves in the back. People with cancer, for example, are usually older or already known to have cancer. They may look ill and have other complaints, like weight loss. Those with infection of the backbone may have fever, infection at some other site, or a medical condition that lowers their immunity. Those with weak bones are prone to breaking the backbone even in the absence of an injury, but it is unlikely in someone of your age. Pressure on the nerves in the back will cause the pain to shoot down the leg, make the legs weak or numb, and cause problems in controlling the waterworks or bowels. Your pain is confined to the back, and your legs are fine, so I don't think there is any pressure on the nerves in the back.*'

He asks what he should do to get better and how long it will take for him to recover.

Outline the management of simple back pain. Tell him that:

- He can take the painkillers prescribed by the ED doctor for symptom relief.

  '*While waiting for the problem to go away, you can take the painkillers prescribed by the doctor who saw you earlier. Those pills can help relax your muscles and reduce the pain. You can also apply a packet of frozen vegetables wrapped in a cloth over your back about three or four times a day to reduce the pain. You can switch to a hot water bottle, again wrapped in a cloth, when the pain starts to subside.*'

- He should remain as active as possible and return to work at the earliest.

  '*Our backbone is supposed to be flexible, so please do not rest for too long. If you rest for too long, the back will become stiffer and delay your recovery. Do not wait for the pain to completely go away before you start moving. You should gradually resume your activities and go back to work as soon as the pain eases. It'll help you recover faster. It may hurt when you start moving, but you won't be damaging your back by doing that.'*

- If symptoms last longer than two weeks, he can see a chiropractor to consider manipulation.

'If your pain does not improve as expected and lasts longer than a couple of weeks, you can see a chiropractor. Chiropractors specialise in problems of the spine. They use their hands to apply force to the muscles and joints of the back and neck.'

He asks if he is at risk of developing ankylosing spondylitis in the future.

- Tell him that his risk of developing ankylosing spondylitis is small, but **the back pain may recur in the future**.

'The back pain may recur in the future, and I am afraid there is nothing much you can do to prevent this. What I do not want you to do is to worry about ankylosing spondylitis every time you develop back pain. As I said earlier, it usually starts during the late teens or early 20s, so your risk of developing it in the future is very small.'

End the conversation by providing advice on what he must do if he is not progressing well. Ask him to seek medical advice if he develops radicular or neurological symptoms in his legs. Tell him that you will provide an information leaflet on the management of simple back pain, or refer him to some useful websites.

In an exam setting, the actor will be asked to accept your explanation if you speak convincingly. In real life, if the patient fails to accept your reassurance and keeps insisting on getting a scan, politely decline. Ordering a scan should be the decision of the doctor and not that of the patient. Remain firm, although it is not always easy. (*'We don't seem to be getting anywhere with this, and I think we should bring this consultation to a close. Please feel free to seek another opinion. If you feel that there is an underlying problem causing your back pain, it'll delay your recovery, and that is exactly what I am trying to prevent.'*) Document the history, examination findings, and your discussion in detail, as you should be able to defend your decision in case he complains.

SUMMARY

This scenario tests your skills in talking to an anxious patient who is demanding a non-indicated scan. You will be expected to:

- Find out more about the back pain and explore his reasons for demanding a scan.
- Reassure him that there are no features to suggest ankylosing spondylitis or other underlying medical conditions that can cause back pain.
- Explain why a scan is not indicated.
- Explain that his presentation is in keeping with simple back pain.

- Guide him on the management of simple back pain, and reassure him about the generally good outcome in a vast majority of patients.
- Allay his anxieties about the risk of developing ankylosing spondylitis in the future.

A variation of this scenario is talking to an anxious patient who is requesting a computed tomography (CT) scan of his chest to screen for lung cancer. He is asymptomatic and has no risk factors. After checking the reason for his request and confirming that he has no symptoms or risk factors for lung cancer, you should tell him that:

- There is insufficient evidence of benefit in screening asymptomatic individuals without risk factors for lung cancer (unlike the situation with bowel, breast, or cervix cancer).

Note: Targeted lung cancer screening with a low-dose CT scan that is being rolled out in England is for people between 55 and 74 years with a history of smoking habit.

- The scan may reveal benign abnormalities, which will lead to further evaluation, like biopsy or follow-up CT scans, thus increasing his anxiety further.

A normal test result may be reassuring, but a false positive result will cause greater anxiety.

- There is a risk of radiation with CT scanning, which by itself is carcinogenic.

Case 29

The 47-Year-Old Man Who Is Demanding Strong Opioids for His Chronic Back Pain

This 47-year-old man presented to the emergency department (ED) earlier this morning with a flare of his long-standing low back pain. The pain has always been localised to the lumbar region, with no radiation down his legs, neurological symptoms in the legs, or sphincter disturbance. There have been no features suggestive of an underlying medical condition, like cancer, infection, or spondylarthritis. Over the years, he has consulted a number of healthcare practitioners, including general practitioners, an orthopaedic surgeon, a chiropractor, and a physiotherapist. He had a magnetic resonance imaging (MRI) scan 18 months ago, which showed degenerative changes in the lumbar spine, with no evidence of nerve root compression.

His background medical problems include diabetes and hyperlipidaemia. He takes codeine, tramadol, and pregabalin for his back pain, having previously tried paracetamol, naproxen, muscle relaxants, amitriptyline, gabapentin, transcutaneous nerve stimulation, acupuncture, and massage. Naproxen caused an allergic skin rash, while none of the other measures were greatly helpful. He smokes about 20 cigarettes a day and drinks a few beers every week. He used to be a train driver but stopped working about two years ago because of his back pain. He lives with his wife.

The ED doctor has asked for your help as he is asking for morphine and she is 'unable to handle his demands'. She feels that his presentation is in keeping with non-specific chronic low back pain. You are the medical registrar in the acute medical unit.

- After the initial introduction, *ask how you can help*.

He says he has had the back pain for a long time but the problem is gradually getting worse. He is fed up because no one is interested in helping him. He hasn't been able to work for nearly two years because of his back pain. He thinks he will end up in a wheelchair one day.

He wants you to prescribe something stronger, like morphine, because the pain has been really bad for the last two to three days. He takes codeine, tramadol, and pregabalin, but they do not afford much relief.

There are several key differences between acute and chronic pain. Acute pain serves a protective function and resolves once the underlying problem is treated ('biomedical approach').

DOI: 10.1201/9781003533337-33

Chronic pain, by comparison, does not serve a protective function (except in a small proportion of patients in whom it is caused by an ongoing medical problem) and persists past the point of tissue healing due to psychosocial factors. The pain is usually accompanied by non-restorative sleep, physical deconditioning, and psychological distress. Management of these patients should also focus on improving physical function and reducing psychological distress ('biopsychosocial approach').

'Yellow flags' (factors that maintain the problem) in chronic back pain include wrong beliefs, passive dependence on practitioners, failure to accept medical reassurance, prolonged absence from work, and unhelpful thoughts, emotions, and behaviours ('*There must be something wrong with my spine*', '*I am fed up*', '*No one is helping me*', '*I will end up in a wheelchair one day*'). Chronic back pain is indeed a very difficult problem to manage, and it may not be possible for a single healthcare practitioner to address all the issues, certainly not in ten minutes. Those with secondary gains because of chronic pain are more challenging because they may not be receptive to your suggestions.

It appears that the main reason for his ED visit was to ask for a stronger analgesic, like morphine. It is important to be mindful of patients with chronic pain whose main problem may be drug dependence or drug-seeking behaviour rather than pain. It should be suspected if the patient (1) sees multiple doctors or visits multiple pharmacies, (2) shows unwillingness to accept other forms of treatment (legitimate sufferers will usually accept your suggestions), (3) grades the pain as 10/10, (4) asks for a specific drug by brand name, or (5) flatters you ('You are my favourite doctor').

- After you say a few reassuring words ('*We are keen to help you*', '*We want you to get better*'), **check his understanding of his back pain** ('*What do you think might be causing your back pain?*').
- *Ask if there is a specific reason for requesting morphine.*

He says he thought his back pain was caused by wear-and-tear changes in his backbone. He asked for morphine as he thought it might be stronger than tramadol or codeine. He is not keen to carry on taking the pills long-term. He is happy to accept any treatment that will take his pain away.

- Tell him that *the degenerative changes seen on the MRI scan will not entirely explain his symptoms.*

  '*The MRI scan done last year indeed showed some wear and tear in your backbone, but these changes will not entirely explain your pain. Wear-and-tear changes are quite common as we grow older. If we scan a hundred people with back pain and another hundred without back pain, we can expect to see such changes in nearly the same proportion of people in both groups.*
  '*I also do not feel that your pain is caused by some medical condition or disease. The idea that all symptoms are caused by disease is incorrect. Symptoms like headache, backache, tingling, constipation, heartburn, and ringing in the ears are quite common but often not caused by a disease. Out of ten people who complain of headache, one or two may be found to have an infection, tumour, or bleeding in the brain. In the rest, the headache is not caused by a disease. They just have a headache. The same is true for back pain as well.*'

Having established that his request for morphine is not due to drug-seeking behaviour:

- **Provide some advice on managing his flares,** which should include pharmacological as well as non-pharmacological measures.

'I'm not very comfortable writing a prescription for morphine. You could become addicted to it and develop side effects, like drowsiness and constipation. I am concerned that we may be doing more harm than good with morphine. If tramadol and codeine are helpful to an extent, I would suggest that you stick with them but without exceeding the recommended dosages.

'In addition to taking painkillers, you can try ice packs or a warm bath. You should start moving as soon as the pain starts to ease, because resting too much will make the muscles stiffer and prolong the flare. You'll feel worse if there is nothing on your mind except the pain, so you should distract yourself as much as possible by doing something that you enjoy, like watching a comedy show, movie, or your favourite sport; listening to music; or reading a book. Flare-ups are quite common in people with long-standing pain. You should think if you did something different during the days preceding the flare and try to avoid them next time.'

- Briefly **ask about his daily routine, sleep, and mood.**

He admits that he has become sedentary ever since he stopped working. He sits on his sofa all day, watching TV or playing games on his phone. His sleep is not good. He wakes up feeling unrefreshed most mornings. He feels a bit low all the time and worries a lot about what might happen to him in the future. His frustration mainly stems from the thought that he must live with this pain for the rest of his life and nothing seems to be working.

Tell him that:

- **Chronic pain will not respond to painkillers alone** and needs a different approach.

'When pain becomes long-standing, it impairs your ability to work, disturbs your sleep, and affects your emotions. Pain, poor sleep, and low mood can aggravate each other and set up a vicious cycle, so pain alone is not the problem anymore. This is the reason you don't find the painkillers helpful.

'We should address each of these elements to make you feel better overall. In addition to reducing the pain, we should look at ways of improving your fitness, sleep, and mood.'

- **It is important to address his unhelpful thoughts, emotions, and behaviours.**

'If you remain convinced that your pain is caused by a medical problem, it'll only increase your distress and make the pain worse. Our thoughts and beliefs can affect our emotions and behaviours in a positive or negative way. In many people, back pain starts as a physical problem, but it becomes persistent and long-standing because of the way they react to the pain, not because the original problem got worse.'

- **He should gradually increase his physical activity.**

'Our backbone is meant to move a lot, so resting too much will make the muscles stiffer and worsen the pain. You should therefore try to gradually increase your physical activity. Start with some gentle walking, and then slowly increase your pace and

distance. It'll make you fitter and reduce the deconditioning – it is one way of breaking the vicious cycle that I talked about just now. It may hurt more when you start moving, but that doesn't mean that you are damaging your backbone.'

He says he understands but is not sure where to start. He asks if there are any medications to improve his sleep and emotions.

- *You will refer him to the multi-disciplinary pain team.*

'I'll prescribe a medication to improve the quality of your sleep and make you feel fresh in the mornings. If that is not helpful on its own, we'll add an antidepressant medication to improve your mood.
'I'll also refer you to our pain team. In addition to doctors who are interested in managing people with long-standing pain, the team includes a psychologist and physiotherapists. The psychologist can address some of your unhelpful thoughts and beliefs, which will help alter the emotions and behaviours in a positive manner. The physiotherapist can help with an exercise program that suits you.'

- *His active involvement is more important than the passive treatments that we offer.*

'Rather than relying on doctors to do everything, it is important for you to take charge and play an active part in self-managing your pain. Gradually increasing your activity, improving your sleep, and changing the way you think or feel about your pain will all help. It may not cure the problem, but even a 50% reduction in pain will make you feel 200% better. As the problem has been there for a long time, it'll take time. I'm afraid there are no quick-fix solutions.'

End the conversation by summarising the main points. Reiterate that (1) his back pain is not caused by an underlying medical condition, (2) it is best to avoid morphine because the benefits do not outweigh its risks, (3) non-pharmacological measures are helpful in managing his flares, and (4) you will prescribe a small dose of amitriptyline and refer him to the pain team.

SUMMARY

This scenario tests your skills in talking to a patient who is demanding strong opioids for his chronic pain problem. You will be expected to:

- Identify his main concerns.
- Make sure he is not requesting morphine because of a drug-seeking behaviour.
- Provide advice on pharmacological and non-pharmacological measures that can help manage his flares.
- Explain that his back pain is not caused by an underlying medical condition.
- Explain that chronic pain needs a multi-disciplinary approach that aims not only to reduce his pain but also to improve his function, sleep, and low mood.
- Tell him that a cure is unrealistic. The overall aim of management is to improve his symptoms and quality of life.

Case 30

The 43-Year-Old Woman with No Diagnosis Despite Extensive Evaluation

This 43-year-old Asian woman was admitted one week ago with a four-week history of fever associated with tiredness and weight loss of about 3–4 kg. Her past medical history is blameless, and she is not taking any regular medication. She denies travelling anywhere recently or keeping any pets at home. She has never knowingly been in contact with anyone with tuberculosis. She does an office-based job. Her family history is unremarkable. She has never smoked or used recreational drugs and drinks alcohol only socially. Her menses are regular. She is in a monogamous relationship with her husband and has two healthy children.

Physical examination over the last week has been unremarkable, except for fever and proportional tachycardia. Investigations done so far have revealed normocytic anaemia, elevated erythrocyte sedimentation rate and C-reactive protein, low serum albumin, low serum iron, and mildly elevated ferritin. Her white cell and platelet counts; peripheral blood film; liver, renal, and thyroid function; serum calcium and phosphate; creatine kinase; lactate dehydrogenase; lipid panel; HbA$_1$c; urinalysis; serum autoantibodies (anti-nuclear antibody, double-stranded antibody, antibodies to extractable antigens, rheumatoid factor, anti-neutrophil cytoplasmic antibody); complement levels; angiotensin-converting enzyme; and myeloma screens are all normal. Three sets of blood cultures have been sterile. Tests for human immunodeficiency virus, hepatitis B and C, COVID-19, Epstein–Barr virus, cytomegalovirus, toxoplasma, brucella, rickettsia, and respiratory virus panel are negative. Chest X-ray; computed tomography scan of the thorax, abdomen, and pelvis; transthoracic echocardiogram; and mammogram are also unremarkable.

She was discussed with the haematologist, rheumatologist, and consultant in infectious diseases yesterday. Their consensus opinion was to ask for a fluorodeoxyglucose positron emission tomography–computed tomography (FDG PET-CT) scan. You are the registrar in the ward. The patient asks you to update her husband, whom you have not met. She says he is quite vexed that you have done numerous tests and still not given them a clear answer.

- Introduce yourself, and confirm the identity of the husband. Tell him that you have come to update him about his wife's progress.

He says he is frustrated that you still haven't told them what the problem is 'even after doing hundreds of blood tests, urine tests, X-rays, and scans'. He asks in an angry tone if you all know what you are doing.

DOI: 10.1201/9781003533337-34

- *Acknowledge his frustration*, and ask what he has been told already.

'We are sorry that we haven't been able to find out the cause of her fever yet. I can understand your frustration. It's frustrating for us too. May I first find out what you have been told so far?'

He says his wife has been going for one test after another ever since she got admitted a week ago. The doctors have been updating him and his wife on a daily basis about the results of the tests. They have so far told them that her inflammation reading is up and she is anaemic. They also told them that the other blood tests, urine tests, CT scan, heart scan, and mammogram are all normal.

Tell him that:

- **The underlying causes of prolonged fever include infection, cancer, and autoimmune disease.**

'In most people with fever, we find a viral or bacterial infection. The fever usually subsides quickly either on its own or with appropriate treatment. In some people, the fever does not subside even after several days or weeks, and we then start thinking of unusual infections, cancers, and autoimmune problems – autoimmune *means the immune system makes a mistake and attacks our own body.'*

- **The investigations done so far have not revealed any of these causes.**

'We had to do multiple tests because her medical history, our examination findings, and the initial tests did not point to the cause of her fever. Regrettably, the second-line tests also did not give us an answer. Although this is disappointing, the important thing is that we haven't found anything serious. There is indeed a small chance that there is something serious, which the tests done so far haven't picked up.'

- **An underlying cause of her fever may never be found.**

'From time to time, we do see people in whom we struggle to make a diagnosis. Sometimes the problem evolves slowly and the diagnosis may only become evident later. In about one in three people with prolonged fever, an underlying cause is never found, and the illness eventually resolves without any treatment.'

He says he is not convinced with your explanation and asks if he could get a second opinion.

- Tell him that **you have discussed with consultants from various specialties.**

'We have discussed her case in detail with various specialists, including a blood specialist; a rheumatologist, who is a specialist on autoimmune problems; and a specialist in infectious diseases. They are experts in dealing with people with prolonged fever.
'You are, of course, free to seek another opinion, but please allow me to share their thoughts with you. [Pause.] All three of them feel that it is best to do a special kind of scan called PET-CT.'

He asks how this scan is better than the ones that you have done already.

- Tell him that *a PET scan can pick up inflammation or cancer much earlier than a CT scan* could.

  'What we did earlier was a CT scan. On a CT scan, we see cancer or inflammation as an abnormal shadow. However, it can take a while before cancer or inflammation shows up on the CT scan. Therefore, we sometimes miss them in the early stages. The advantage of a PET scan is that it can show the cancer or inflammation at a much earlier stage compared to a CT scan.'

- Briefly *explain how the PET-CT scan works.*

  'The PET-CT scan is two different scans combined into one. They'll first inject a special sugar substance into the vein. The sugar will get into all the cells and emit a small amount of radiation. If there are cancer cells or inflammatory cells, they'll take up more sugar than the other cells and give out more radiation. We can see the parts of the body that are emitting more radiation as bright spots on the scan.

  'We then have the option of taking a sample of cells from the part of the body that is emitting more radiation and sending it to the lab so that it can be examined under the microscope. We call this biopsy. A PET scan is also better than the other types of scans to detect some unusual causes of prolonged fever, like inflammation of the muscles or the lining of the blood vessels.'

He asks if this scan will definitely give an answer and why it was not done earlier.

- Tell him that *there is no guarantee that the PET-CT scan will give us an answer.* It was not considered earlier as it is not a first-line investigation.

  'We did not ask for this scan earlier because it is not a first-line test. We ask for this scan only if the other tests do not give us an answer. I am afraid this scan may or may not give us an answer. However, if it is completely normal, there is a very high chance that her illness will resolve in due course.'

He says he is concerned that you are injecting a substance that emits radiation into her body.

- *Discuss the risks of a PET-CT scan.*

  'There is no radiation risk from the sugar substance. The sugar should be flushed out of the body by the end of the day. She should just avoid being very close to pregnant women or young children for a few hours after having the scan.

  'There is, however, some radiation risk from the CT, which is the second part of the scan. In a small number of people, the dye used with the CT scan can cause an allergic reaction or harm the kidneys. Harm to the kidneys is more common in people with pre-existing kidney problems. It is unlikely that she'll have these reactions, as her kidneys are working well and we have already used that dye when she had the earlier scans.'

He says his uncle is a retired GP. He suggested that steroids should be tried to control the fever. He asks if you would consider that.

Tell him that:

- *PET-CT is a better option than empirical steroid therapy.*

    'We used to blindly give steroids after ruling out infections, but it was before the days when PET-CT scans were available. Steroids are probably still tried in parts of the world where these scans are not widely available. If we start steroids, we might have to deal with the side effects of steroids, like a rise in blood pressure and blood sugar, weight gain, and thinning of bones. Moreover, we wouldn't know what we are treating, so the initial dose of steroid, how long to treat, and how to lower the dose will all be based on guess-work. We would therefore not recommend giving her steroids, at least for now.'

- *If the PET-CT is normal, you would prefer to continue to observe her.*

    'People with prolonged fever are sometimes subjected to invasive procedures, like biopsies from the bone marrow, which is the inner part of the bone, or an operation to open the tummy to check for any infection. In countries where tuberculosis is common, doctors start medications for tuberculosis even if the test results are normal.
    'In her case, if the PET-CT is normal, and as long as fever is the only issue, I think we should sit on the fence and continue to observe.'

End the discussion by reassuring him that you will make sure she is not subjected to any unnecessary tests. Tell him that you will continue to liaise with the specialists and regularly update them. He and his wife can discuss and let them know their decision regarding getting the PET-CT scan, but they are free to seek a second opinion if they wish to do so.

SUMMARY

This scenario tests your skills in talking to a frustrated husband about the inability to reach a diagnosis in his wife, who continues to spike a fever. You will be expected to:

- Acknowledge the husband's frustration.
- Explain why so many tests had to be done.
- Tell him that an underlying cause of PUO is sometimes never found.
- Tell him that he is free to seek a second opinion.
- Share with him the opinions of the different specialists with whom her case was discussed.
- Explain why the team wishes to do a PET-CT and how this is different from the scans that she has already had.
- Explain why you wouldn't recommend empirical steroid therapy yet.

The 66-Year-Old Man Whose Sister Does Not Agree with Your Diagnosis

This 66-year-old man with a background history of diabetes mellitus and hyperlipidaemia presented to the emergency department (ED) yesterday (it was a Saturday) with a four-week history of pain around his shoulders and hips associated with early morning stiffness lasting a few hours. His younger sister, who works abroad as a urology nurse practitioner, came to visit him a couple of days ago. She chided him for not seeking medical advice earlier and decided to bring him to the ED.

He denied headache, visual symptoms, jaw claudication, loss of weight, night sweats, or swelling in his joints. Systems enquiry was entirely unremarkable. His vital signs were normal, and physical examination was unremarkable. His erythrocyte sedimentation rate (ESR) was 92 mm/hour, and C-reactive protein (CRP) 64 mg/L. His blood counts; glucose, liver, and renal function; HbA$_1$c; urinalysis; and chest X-ray were normal. Although the ED physician was keen on arranging an urgent outpatient appointment, the sister demanded admission.

You saw him earlier today in the ward with your consultant, who diagnosed polymyalgia rheumatica (PMR). She explained the diagnosis to him and suggested oral prednisolone. The patient, however, asked the consultant to discuss the diagnosis and treatment plan with his sister later. It is now 4:00 p.m. on a Sunday, and his sister has just arrived. The consultant has left the site, and you are the registrar on call. The ward nurse has informed you that she wishes to speak to the medical team about her brother. She warns you that "she is a bit difficult".

- Introduce yourself. Confirm her identity and her relationship to the patient.

In real life, always take a chaperone when you go see such 'difficult' relatives.

She confirms that she is his sister, but in response to your questions on whether she is a nurse practitioner and where she works, she replies curtly, 'Why does it matter to you what job I do or where I work? It's not about me. We are here to talk about my brother. Let's stick to that. Where's your consultant by the way?'

DOI: 10.1201/9781003533337-35

- Remain calm and conduct yourself professionally. *Tell her that you would be happy to answer any questions that she may have.*

'I saw your brother with my consultant this morning. She'll be back tomorrow morning. I am happy to update you about your brother and answer as many of your questions as possible. Before I start, may I ask what exactly your concerns are?'

She continues to talk in an angry tone and says she does not agree with your diagnosis. She is worried about infection, as his ESR and CRP are so high. She feels that the team should do blood cultures and start him on antibiotics. She says she is appalled that a 66-year-old diabetic man with such a high ESR and CRP has been sent to the general ward and not the high-dependency unit.

This woman comes across as hostile, confrontational, and unpleasant, with some misconceptions and unreasonable demands. Indeed, we all regularly come across such unreasonable patients or relatives, whose requests may range from asking for extended medical certificates and unnecessary specialist referrals for trivial issues to non-indicated diagnostic tests or treatments. Dealing with such individuals requires patience, skill, and experience.

The challenge here is that PMR is a clinical diagnosis that is made on the basis of symptoms and elevated inflammatory markers. However, elevated ESR and CRP are not specific to PMR, and there are no confirmatory laboratory, radiological, or histological studies. A rapid response to corticosteroid is the best way to confirm the diagnosis. All this should be clearly explained to her. She should also be told that his elevated inflammatory markers are unlikely to be due to infection.

- Explain why *you feel that his presentation is in keeping with PMR.*

'I can see that you are upset. Please allow me to explain. Polymyalgia is essentially an inflammatory condition that affects people over the age of 50. It causes pain and stiffness of the muscles around the shoulders and hips. Symptoms are worse first thing in the morning, and they gradually ease as the day progresses. These are the exact symptoms that your brother has been experiencing for the last month or so, which is why we thought of it.'

- Tell her that *the elevated ESR and CRP would support a diagnosis of PMR* in the context of his clinical presentation.

'We often see a high ESR or CRP in people with polymyalgia, so that fits in as well. I appreciate your concern, but a high ESR or CRP is not specific to infection – they also go up in people with any form of inflammation. We always consider the overall clinical presentation when we interpret the ESR or CRP. We never look at the test results in isolation.'

She asks if you have done any tests to confirm that his pain is due to polymyalgia and how you can be so sure that his elevated ESR and CRP are due to polymyalgia before ruling out an infection.

- Tell her that *the diagnosis was considered on the basis of his overall clinical presentation.*

'I am afraid there is no specific test to confirm the diagnosis of polymyalgia. We considered it on the basis of his symptoms and the high ESR and CRP.

'Polymyalgia responds beautifully to steroid pills. The symptoms usually vanish within two to three days of starting the steroid. The ESR and CRP should also fall soon after starting the steroid. Therefore, the best way to confirm the diagnosis of polymyalgia is to assess his response to steroid pills – see whether the symptoms resolve and the ESR and CRP fall.'

Aren't steroids dangerous in case he has an undiagnosed infection? she asks.

Tell her that:

- *His overall presentation does not support a diagnosis of infection.*

'We feel that his overall presentation does not support a diagnosis of infection. An infection is unlikely to present with pain and stiffness confined to the shoulders and hips for so many weeks. Moreover, there are no symptoms to suggest an infection, like fever, sweats, weight loss, headache, skin rashes, swollen joints, cough, breathlessness, abdominal pain, diarrhoea, or painful urination.

'His vital signs have been stable, and we did not find any abnormal signs when we examined him. His chest X-ray is normal, the urine is clear, and the rest of his results, including the liver and kidney function, are all normal. All this is reassuring. In the absence of clear evidence of infection, we do not feel that there is a need to do blood cultures or start him on antibiotics.'

- *If he agrees, he will be commenced on a moderate dose of prednisolone.* The necessary precautions will be taken to minimise the side effects.

'Steroids are indeed associated with side effects, like a rise in blood pressure and blood sugar, weight gain, and osteoporosis, but it depends on the dose and duration of treatment. The larger the dose of steroid and the longer the duration of treatment, the higher the risk of getting side effects.

'For polymyalgia, we start a moderate dose of steroids, usually around 20 mg of prednisolone. We'll refer him to a rheumatologist, who will monitor his progress and gradually taper the dose over several months. It'll hopefully help minimise the side effects. We'll be taking a few more precautions – we'll screen him for hepatitis B, check his vitamin D level, arrange a bone density scan, and give him the flu and pneumococcal shots, if he hasn't had them already.'

- *It is possible that he may not respond to the steroid.*

'There is a very good chance that he will respond to the prednisolone, but there is also a small chance that he may not respond to it, in which case we'll revisit the diagnosis. It's certainly not a diagnosis written on stone, but right now, it seems like the most likely one. The rheumatologist will discuss the next steps if there is no response to the steroid.'

She insists on seeing the consultant before he is commenced on steroid. She says she wants to see her straightaway. She is not happy that you are starting him on a dangerous medication for a diagnosis that cannot be proved by blood tests, X-rays, or scans.

Tell her that:

- *You do not intend to start him on steroids that evening.*

   '*We won't be starting the steroids tonight and certainly not without your brother's consent. It can wait until tomorrow morning. Steroids will not work straightaway. It'll take two or three days to start working, so there is no rush to start them tonight.*'

- *The consultant will see him the following morning.*

   '*As he is stable, my consultant will see him tomorrow morning. I'm afraid there is nothing further for her to add to what I have just told you. Being a healthcare worker yourself, you may be well aware that senior physician presence is not possible around the clock except in places like the emergency department or intensive care unit. The surgeons and those who perform procedures like cardiologists and gastroenterologists also leave the site after office hours and come back only if they are called for an emergency. I'd like to reassure you that the team here on the site has the necessary skills to manage the full range of emergencies. We'll take advice from our consultant over the phone if needed.*'

If she keeps insisting:

- Remain firm and end the conversation by saying that you will get the consultant to speak to her the following morning.

   '*I have tried my best to explain why we think infection is unlikely and antibiotics are not indicated. I'll get my consultant to speak to you tomorrow morning in the presence of your brother. I certainly do not wish to do something that is likely to cause harm or not help.*'

In real life, do not forget to go back and talk to the brother, because he is the patient, not her ('*Because of some reservations expressed by your sister, I will arrange for the consultant to talk to both of you in the morning*'). There is no need to tell him that she was difficult or aggressive. Reassure him that the decision to start steroid can wait until the following morning.

This is a scenario that gives a chance for the consultant (examiner) to see how you would deal with a difficult relative in the middle of the night! When dealing with angry or upset patients or relatives, (1) you must listen to their concerns, (2) acknowledge their anger ('*I can see that you are upset*'), (3) ask why they are upset, (4) try to see their point of view, and (5) apologise if there was any error. Do not try to dominate the consultation or be dismissive. It is important to find a balance between not forcing your opinion on them and, at the same time, not yielding to their unreasonable demands.

If there is a threat of physical or verbal abuse, the security personnel should be alerted and the matter brought to the attention of the patient liaison service. Make it clear that abuse will not be tolerated. ('*I cannot let you talk to me in that tone or manner. I find your behaviour and language unacceptable. I am afraid I'll have to call the security personnel to assist me. We have a right to work without being abused, intimidated, or threatened.'*)

SUMMARY

This scenario tests your skills in talking to a difficult relative who challenges your diagnosis. You will be expected to:

- Listen to her concerns.
- Remain calm and conduct yourself professionally.
- Explain that his presentation is in keeping with PMR and there are no clinical pointers to infection.
- Clear her misconceptions about ESR and CRP.

Tell her that elevated ESR and CRP may be encountered in any inflammatory condition and are not specific to infection.

- Discuss the rationale for suggesting treatment with corticosteroid.
- Show humility. Tell her that if steroids prove unhelpful, the diagnosis will be revisited.
- Gently turn down her request to see the consultant on a Sunday evening.

Do not force your opinion on her or yield to her unreasonable demands.

When Things Go Wrong

The 68-Year-Old Man Whose Stroke Was Not Diagnosed in Time

This 68-year-old man presented to the emergency department (ED) two days ago with vertigo. He denied weakness or numbness in his limbs and face, unsteadiness of gait, visual loss, diplopia, slurred speech, headache, hearing loss, or tinnitus. His background medical problems included hypertension and hyperlipidaemia, for which he took amlodipine and atorvastatin every day. He smoked for a few years during his 20s, but never since then, and drank alcohol only during weekends.

Physical examination was unremarkable, with no focal neurological deficits or cerebellar signs. His vertigo was diagnosed as 'peripheral', and he was treated with β-histine and prochlorperazine. He was discharged home the following morning as he reported marked improvement in his vertigo. An outpatient appointment was arranged in the otology clinic.

Twenty-four hours after the patient went home, his vertigo suddenly got worse, accompanied by unsteadiness of gait and slurring of speech. His wife brought him back to the ED straightaway. Computed tomography (CT) scan of the brain revealed a large cerebellar infarct. He was given a loading dose of aspirin, but thrombolysis was not considered, as he was past the time window.

Two hours after admission, his Glasgow Coma Scale (GCS) dropped to 10/15. His other vital parameters remained stable, with blood pressure around 140/90 mmHg and oxygen saturation of 95% on room air. The repeat CT scan showed cerebellar oedema around the infarct. He was therefore urgently shifted to the intensive care unit (ICU) and given mannitol to reduce intracranial tension (ICT). He has been referred to the neurosurgeon for an opinion on whether an external ventricular drain or operative decompression is required to reduce the risk of brainstem compression.

It is now 7:00 p.m., and the daughter has just arrived. You are the medical registrar on call. Your task is to explain the diagnosis and management plan to her.

- Introduce yourself, and check her identity and relationship to the patient. *Ask what she has been told already.*

The daughter looks upset. She says she brought her father to the hospital two days ago as he complained of giddiness. The doctors discharged him yesterday after telling them that the giddiness was due to some fluid imbalance in the inner part of the ear and it was not serious.

DOI: 10.1201/9781003533337-37

She heard from her mother that his giddiness got worse this morning and he was suddenly not able to walk or talk properly. She is very disappointed, because she feels that he was discharged hastily during his previous admission.

Tell her that:

- *Her father has suffered a stroke.*

   'I can see that you are upset. I'll talk about his previous admission in a short while. Let me first tell you how he is at present. We arranged a brain scan as soon as he arrived because he was unable to walk steadily and his speech was slurred. I'm afraid the scan showed a stroke affecting the rear end of the brain. A stroke occurs when a blood clot forms in a blood vessel supplying the brain. It cuts off the blood supply to that part of the brain.'

- *He was given an anti-platelet agent.*

   'We gave him a blood-thinning tablet right away to prevent further blood clots from forming and making the stroke larger.'

The daughter says she is dismayed. She never expected his giddiness to turn out to be due to something so serious. She asks why her father has been shifted from the general ward to the intensive care unit.

- Tell her that he was shifted to the ICU because *his GCS dropped and the CT scan showed cerebellar oedema.*

   'He was fully alert at the time of admission, but a couple of hours later, he became less conscious. We repeated the scan of his brain, and it showed fluid collection in the brain. The pressure in his brain was high because of the fluid collection. It is one of the complications that we see in people with stroke. We have shifted him to the intensive care unit so that he can be closely monitored.'

- *Tell her how he is being managed in the ICU.*

   'A very high pressure in the brain can sometimes cause an injury to the brainstem, which is the part of the brain that controls our breathing and blood pressure. We have given him a medication to quickly reduce the pressure in the brain. We have asked a brain surgeon to see him. He might suggest inserting a tube into the space inside the brain to drain some of the fluid and reduce the pressure, or even consider an operation. He'll talk to you after he has seen him.'

- Tell her that *he will be closely monitored in the ICU.*

   'I'm afraid your father is quite unwell at the moment. We'll continue to monitor him closely. He will need the support of a breathing machine if his conscious level drops further or the brainstem is affected because of the high pressure in the brain.'

🗨 At this stage, it is sufficient to give her some basic information about (1) her father's diagnosis (stroke), (2) the complication that he has suffered (cerebellar oedema), (3) what has been done so far (loaded with aspirin, transferred to ICU, given mannitol), (4) the next steps (close monitoring, neurosurgical opinion), and (5) his prognosis (he is unwell and may need the support of a ventilator). There is no need to discuss his long-term management or measures that are aimed at preventing a further stroke (e.g. higher dose of statin, echocardiogram to look for a cardioembolic source, rehabilitation, general lifestyle measures).

She asks if the outcome would have been different if he had been scanned when he was brought to the hospital the first time or at least kept in the hospital for a longer period of time. She wonders if any early signs of stroke were missed during his earlier admission.

🗨 You should have anticipated this question even before you walked into the room! While it is important to be open and honest, you should bear in mind that it is difficult to answer this question without hearing 'the other side of the story' from the team that managed him during the previous admission. You can tell her that you will ask the previous medical team to talk to her. You should not be too defensive or dismissive, use medicolegal terms that cannot be retracted later (e.g. '*I am sorry that we were negligent*'), or blame your colleagues.

Explain the difficulties in diagnosing posterior circulation stroke. Tell her that:

- Vertigo could be due to a peripheral or central cause.

  '*The giddiness your father experienced – we call this vertigo – may be caused by a problem in the inner part of the ear, which is not so serious, or a problem in the brain, which is commonly due to a stroke.*'

- It is often difficult to diagnose stroke when patients present with vertigo alone without other manifestations (without sounding too defensive).

  '*In people with vertigo, it is often difficult to know for sure if it is due to a problem in the ear or the brain, especially when there are no other symptoms to suggest a stroke. Stroke affecting the front part of the brain often presents with clear-cut symptoms, like weakness, numbness, slurred speech, or sudden loss of eyesight, making it relatively easier to diagnose it early.*
  '*Stroke affecting the rear end of the brain, on the other hand, is not so straightforward. From what I can gather from his notes, he did not report any other symptom apart from giddiness, and the team that managed your father did not find any signs of stroke when they examined him. We do not scan everyone with giddiness.*'

- It is difficult to say if the outcome might have been different.

  '*If he had been scanned during his previous admission and the stroke had been diagnosed early, we could have possibly given him a medication to dissolve the blood clot. The outcome of stroke is indeed better if the clot is dissolved early. However, this medication must be given within 4 1/2 hours from the onset of symptoms.*
  '*It is often difficult to achieve this in people with stroke affecting the rear end of the brain. We usually do a CT scan in the emergency department, which often does*

not show the stroke at the rear end of the brain in the early stage. Another type of scan called MRI is better to diagnose this kind of stroke early, but the MRI scan is not widely available in the emergency setting. The medication that dissolves the blood clot can increase the risk of bleeding, so we don't give it unless we find definite evidence of stroke on the scan.'

- In hindsight, it appears that he either had a transient ischaemic attack or his stroke was possibly in evolution when he presented the first time.

'The team probably decided to discharge him as his giddiness improved and there were no other features pointing to stroke. In hindsight, it appears that his stroke was slowly developing at that time or he possibly had what we call a mini-stroke. In a mini-stroke, the blood vessel gets blocked by a blood clot but the clot dissolves on its own after a while, thus restoring the blood flow to the brain. I'll ask the doctors who managed your father during the previous admission to talk to you. I do not wish to say too much without hearing their thoughts.'

She says she might ask for a copy of his medical notes to check if he was evaluated properly and examined thoroughly the first time. She still feels that a man of his age, with high blood pressure and high cholesterol, who was at high risk of developing a stroke, should not have been discharged within a day. She would soon be speaking to her cousin, who is a lawyer.

Tell her that:
- *Due process will be followed if the family wishes to look at his medical notes.*

'Your father, of course, has the right to ask for a copy of his medical notes, but he is not in a state to do so at present. If he does not regain his ability to make decisions for himself, there is a process to follow for his relatives to ask for the notes. I'll ask the relevant people to discuss with you regarding this request.'

- *A full investigation will be conducted.*

'I am sorry you are going through this. We will certainly investigate this thoroughly and share the findings with you. Right now, let's focus on getting him well. The doctors in the intensive care unit will keep you updated of his progress.'

Note: Offering an apology is not an admission of liability, but do not say, 'I am sorry you feel that way' (which might be perceived as a bit rude, implying that there is no mistake on your part), or 'I am sorry we missed the stroke' (which you cannot say without a full investigation).

The patient has a right to ask for a copy of his medical notes in case he wishes to gather evidence to make a complaint about his healthcare. He does not have to give a reason for wanting to see his records. If the patient lacks capacity, his healthcare attorney with lasting power of attorney (LPA), or the court-appointed deputy (CAD), can ask for the notes. Any information that is likely to cause physical or mental harm, or confidential information about someone else, can be withheld before releasing the records. If the person lacks capacity and there is no LPA or CAD, the matter should be discussed with the ethics committee and the medical director. It should be possible to take a decision in the best interests of the patient and release the relevant parts of the notes to the next of kin in most cases.

SUMMARY

This scenario tests your skills in talking to a family member about a diagnostic delay that results in a serious outcome. You will be expected to:

- Explain his current clinical state and management plans in layman's terms (diagnosis, treatments provided so far, the next steps, prognosis).
- Acknowledge her anger and frustration.
- Explain the possible reasons for the delayed diagnosis without being too defensive.
- State only the facts, not your assumptions or personal opinions.
- Tell her that you will ask the previous team to talk to her.

Do not push the blame to the previous team, and do not let out any medicolegal terms that cannot be retracted later.

- Tell her that a full investigation will be conducted and the findings shared with her.
- If she asks, tell her that she is free to make a complaint, and reassure her that it will not affect the care of her father.

A variation of this case is talking to the husband of a young woman with a background history of asthma who presented to the emergency department two days ago with a one-day history of breathlessness. She denied wheezing, chest pain, cough, or haemoptysis. Her asthma was well controlled, and she seldom used her inhaler. Her heart rate was 100/minute, but the rest of the vital parameters, including oxygen saturation, were normal.

Her examination was unremarkable. Her chest X-ray, 12-lead electrocardiogram, full blood count, renal function, and thyroid-stimulating hormone were normal. Urine pregnancy test was negative. She was admitted overnight for observation. Although her heart rate remained high at around 90–100/minute, she was discharged the following morning as she reported significant improvement in her symptoms. She was told that her symptoms were most likely due to mild asthma exacerbation or viral bronchitis.

She has now re-presented several hours later, with worsening breathlessness and dizziness. Her vital parameters on arrival showed heart rate 110/minute, blood pressure 80/50 mmHg, respiratory rate 30/min, and oxygen saturation 90% on room air. An urgent bedside echocardiogram has revealed right ventricular dilatation with reduced systolic function and flattening of the interventricular septum, in keeping with massive pulmonary embolism. She has been shifted to the intensive care unit and commenced on high-flow oxygen, intravenous fluid bolus, unfractionated heparin, and inotropes. As she is too unwell for computed tomographic pulmonary angiography, the decision has been taken to commence intravenous tissue plasminogen on clinical grounds.

When talking to the husband, you should follow the same approach that is outlined for the patient with delayed diagnosis of stroke.

The 74-Year-Old Woman Who Has Suffered Harm Because of a Medication Error

This 74-year-old woman, with a background history of hypertension, diabetes mellitus, hyperlipidaemia, heart failure with reduced ejection fraction, and non-alcoholic fatty liver disease, was admitted three days ago with a productive cough and breathlessness. She was diagnosed with community-acquired pneumonia and acute decompensated heart failure. She was commenced on oxygen by nasal prongs, amoxicillin–clavulanic acid, azithromycin, and furosemide.

She was clinically improving, and her vital parameters remained satisfactory. However, she suddenly developed dizziness and palpitations earlier this morning. Her heart rate was 150/minute and blood pressure 106/78 mmHg at that time. Her 12-lead electrocardiogram showed torsades de pointes. She was given intravenous magnesium sulphate, following which her symptoms resolved rapidly, and the rhythm reverted to normal. Her corrected QT (QTc) interval was noted to be 580 ms (normal <440 ms). She was commenced on oral potassium replacement, as her serum potassium was 3.3 mmol/L (normal 3.5–5 mmol/L). Serum magnesium and troponin were normal.

It was only realised after this event that her QTc on admission was already prolonged at 520 ms, and azithromycin was erroneously prescribed and given for two days. Azithromycin has now been discontinued. Her vital parameters are stable at present, but the plan is to shift her to a ward with continuous cardiac monitoring facility because of the risk of recurrence of torsades.

The patient has asked the medical team to update her daughter. You are the medical registrar. Your task is to talk to her daughter about the drug error and the next steps.

Torsades de pointes literally means 'twisting of the points'. It is so named as the QRS complexes appear twisted around the isoelectric line. A prolonged QT interval (interval between onset of depolarisation and completion of repolarisation) is a risk factor for torsades. As the QT interval varies with the heart rate, it is corrected for the heart rate and reported as QTc. A QTc of >500 ms increases the risk of torsades and ventricular arrythmia. It can potentially degenerate into ventricular fibrillation and cause death.

A prolonged QTc is usually caused by drugs (e.g. macrolides, quinolones, chlorpromazine, tricyclic antidepressants, lithium) or electrolyte disturbances (e.g. hypokalaemia, hypomagnesaemia). It may be asymptomatic or present with dizziness and syncope. The treatment of

DOI: 10.1201/9781003533337-38

torsades is intravenous magnesium sulphate (even in patents with normal serum magnesium), correction of serum electrolytes, and removal of the offending agent. Some patients may need isoprenaline or transvenous pacing to accelerate the heart rate. Torsades often terminates spontaneously, but it frequently recurs if the underlying cause is not corrected. Prognosis is excellent, and no long-term treatment is required once the QTc interval returns to normal.

Patients often lose trust in their healthcare providers when errors happen, but the manner in which we respond and the timeliness of the response can have a profound impact on the likelihood of restoring trust. Patients or relatives usually expect three things from the health-care provider: (1) a sincere apology (a bad apology is worse than no apology at all), (2) a clear narration of the events that led to the error, and (3) an outline of the steps that will be taken to avoid similar errors in the future. Make sure you cover these three issues during your conversation with her. There may be an offer of a financial compensation for any harm that has been done, but there is no need to discuss that at this stage.

- Introduce yourself, and confirm her identity and relationship to the patient. *Ask what she has been told so far.*

She says she was told that her mother's breathing trouble was due to a combination of infection and excess fluid in the lungs. She is aware that she is on antibiotics and a water tablet to remove the excess fluid. She is pleased that she is getting better. She is hoping that she can be discharged home soon.

- Tell her that *her mother has responded well to antibiotics and the diuretic.*

'She has indeed responded well to the treatments. She has no fever, and her pulse, breathing, oxygen level in the blood, and blood pressure are all normal. She must continue taking the water tablet and complete the antibiotic course.'

- Ask if her mother told her what happened earlier that morning.

She says she was going to ask you about it. Her mother told her that she suddenly became dizzy and felt her heart racing. It only lasted a short while. She felt fine after a medicine was given through her vein. She asks if it was anything to be concerned about.

Tell her that:

- *Her mother developed a cardiac arrhythmia.*

'Yes, she suddenly complained of dizziness this morning and felt her heart racing. The tracing of her heart at that time showed that her heartbeat was fast and irregular. After we gave her the appropriate treatment, the heartbeat quickly returned to normal within a few minutes.
'An electrical signal passes through the heart muscle to make the heart pump blood. A slowing of this signal along the path can cause this kind of an irregular heartbeat. If it is not treated promptly, it can even stop the heart. Thankfully, she responded well to the treatment that we administered.'

- *She has been commenced on oral potassium replacement,* as serum levels were found to be low.

'Her blood tests done at that time showed that her potassium level was a bit low. A low potassium level can cause this kind of irregular heartbeat. The water tablet that she is taking can cause the potassium level to go down. We are now giving her potassium tablets to replace it.'

After a brief pause, tell her that:

- *You would like to tell her about a mistake that contributed to this problem.*

'I would like to tell you about a mistake that we made which may have contributed to this problem. The tracing of the heart done at the time of admission already showed the slowing of the electrical signal. We avoid giving certain medications in people with this kind of slowing. Azithromycin, one of the two antibiotics that we had been giving her to treat the lung infection, is one of them.

'We overlooked the slowing of the electrical signal on the tracing and gave this antibiotic by mistake. We suspect it further slowed the electrical signal and triggered the irregular heartbeat. It could have been life-threatening, but thankfully, she responded to the treatment that we gave her and the heartbeat quickly returned to normal. We are so sorry that we made this mistake.'

She is taken aback upon hearing this. She asks how long she was given the antibiotic that triggered the irregular heartbeat.

- Tell her that *azithromycin was given for two days and it has now been discontinued.*

'The antibiotic was given once daily for two days – the day before yesterday and yesterday. The usual course is three days, but we have stopped it now.

'She can continue taking Augmentin, the other antibiotic. We had to start her on two different antibiotics as there are some bacteria that do not respond to Augmentin.'

She says this is completely unacceptable. She asks in an angry tone if her mother's heart will be permanently damaged because of the antibiotic.

- Tell her that *once the QTc interval returns to normal, there are no long-term consequences.*

'She is at risk of developing the irregular heartbeat again until the slowing of the electrical signal is corrected. We therefore plan to shift her to another ward so that her heart tracing can be monitored continuously. Once the tracing returns to normal, there are no long-term consequences. It is not a permanent problem. There won't be any damage to the heart because of this.'

She says that while she appreciates you for being honest and admitting the mistake, she is appalled that the team was so careless. She asks you to name the person who prescribed the antibiotic.

Tell her that:

- *You are unable to single out anyone in particular.*

  '*I agree that this is not acceptable at all. We sincerely apologise for this oversight. I do not wish to offer any excuses for the mistake. We always check the heart tracing before prescribing this antibiotic, but we somehow failed to do that on this occasion. I am unable to single out anyone, however. It was a collective error made by the team. Our whole team will take responsibility for this mistake.*'

- *You will be submitting an incident report.*

  '*We will thoroughly investigate to find out what went wrong and put in corrective measures in place so that this mistake is not repeated. We'll learn from this mistake and make sure the message is conveyed to the other doctors. Once we complete the investigations, we'll let you know what we found and how we will prevent this mistake in the future.*'

'You will, of course, defend your colleague, so there is no point in asking you', she says. She continues to talk in an angry tone and wonders if those who made this mistake were qualified enough to take care of patients. She comments that her mother is not a guinea pig for them to learn by making a mistake on her. She asks if she can make a complaint.

- Tell her that *she can make a complaint and this will not affect the care of her mother.*

  '*You can indeed make a complaint. I'll give you the contact details of the patient liaison service department. Regardless of whether or not you proceed with the complaint, we will thoroughly investigate the problem to find out what went wrong. Making a complaint will not affect the care of your mother in any way.*'

End the discussion by summarising the main points. Apologise once again, and tell her that her mother will soon be shifted to another ward so that she can be monitored closely. If all is well, she should be able to go home in a few days. Tell her that if she has any further queries, you would be happy to come back and talk to her.

SUMMARY

This scenario tests your skills in talking to a relative about a medication error that led to patient harm. You will be expected to:

- Provide an update to the daughter on the progress of her mother.
- Make a disclosure about the medication error, and sincerely apologise for the oversight.
- Clearly explain what went wrong and how she is being managed.
- Reassure her that there won't be any long-term consequences to the heart.

- Tell her that the whole team will take responsibility for the error. Do not single out anyone.
- Tell her that an incident report will be submitted, and measures will be put in place so that this error is not repeated.
- Tell her that if she makes a complaint, it will not affect the care of her mother.

Variations of this scenario may include errors with other medications such as insulin (e.g. administering the wrong preparation or dosage, resulting in hypoglycaemia), antibiotics (e.g. overlooking an allergy), and anticoagulants (e.g. prescribing the incorrect dose, resulting in bleeding).

The 78-Year-Old Man Who Fell Off His Bed in the Ward

This 78-year-old man, with a background history of Alzheimer's dementia, stroke, and hypertension, was admitted four days ago with increasing confusion. He was diagnosed with pneumonia and commenced on antibiotics. As he was deemed to be at increased risk of falls, appropriate precautions were taken, which included raising the bed rails, having a call light at the bedside, and placing his possessions within his reach. He was improving clinically, and his mental state slowly seemed to be reaching his baseline.

He unfortunately fell off his bed a short while ago. At the time when he fell, one of the two nurses in his bay was attending to another patient, and the other nurse had just gone to pick something up from the nursing counter. He probably tried to climb over the bed rail, but it was not clear why he did that. He did not seem restless or agitated when he was last seen by the nurses about 15 minutes before he fell. After he fell, he was seen by the junior doctor straightaway. There was a 5 cm laceration over the forehead and some bruising around the right eye. An urgent computed tomography (CT) scan of the brain was arranged, which showed a small subdural haematoma on the right side. There was no skull fracture. The laceration was sutured, and aspirin was withheld. He was discussed with the neurosurgeon, who did not feel that operative intervention was indicated. He suggested monitoring his Glasgow Coma Scale (GCS) and repeating the CT scan if there was a drop in his GCS. His vital parameters and GCS (14/15, which is his baseline) have been stable since the fall.

His daughter has just arrived on the ward. She has not seen her father yet, as he has been taken down to the eye clinic. You are the medical registrar. Your task is to let her know that her father fell in the ward and discuss the next steps.

- Introduce yourself, and confirm her identity and relationship to the patient.

She wonders why you have come to speak to her now, as another doctor from the team updated her this morning over the phone and told her that her father was responding well to the treatment.

DOI: 10.1201/9781003533337-39

- *Tell her what happened.*

'Your father is indeed responding well to the antibiotics. I am here to talk to you about something else. I am very sorry, but this is going to be difficult. [Pause.] A short while ago, your father fell off the bed and hit his head.'

She starts screaming and says this is completely unacceptable. She asks how he is and why he is not on his bed.

- *Tell her how he is at present and how he was managed after the fall.*

'He is stable at present. He is no more confused than usual. The rest of his parameters, including pulse, blood pressure, breathing, and oxygen level in the blood, are all normal. He developed a bruise around his right eye, so we have sent him to the eye clinic to get his eyes checked. He sustained a cut on his forehead, which we have sutured. It was about 5 centimetres long.

'We did an urgent scan of his head, and it showed a small collection of blood around his brain on the right side. There was no fracture of any of his skull bones.'

'Blood around his brain!' she exclaims. She asks if he is going to be OK and what you are going to do about the bleeding in the brain.

Tell her that:

- *The neurosurgeon did not feel that operative intervention was necessary.*

'We consulted the brain surgeon. He did not feel that an operation was necessary to remove the blood clot. We've stopped the aspirin, the blood-thinning tablet that he was taking, as it can make the bleeding worse. If he remains stable, we'll restart the aspirin at a later date, after consulting the brain surgeon.'

- *You will continue to monitor him closely.*

'We will continue to monitor him closely. If he becomes less conscious or more confused, we'll repeat the brain scan to check if the blood clot around the brain is increasing in size. We are hoping that he will remain stable and the blood clot will dissolve soon.'

She continues to talk in an angry tone. She asks how he could have fallen when so many of you were around. She feels that he must have fallen because the staff on the floor were irresponsible.

- Tell her that *appropriate precautions were taken to prevent him from falling*.

'It appears that he tried to climb over the bed rail before he fell off the bed and landed on the floor. We took appropriate precautions to prevent him from falling. We raised his bed rails, placed his possessions within his reach, and gave him a call light to use if he wanted anything.

'He was responding well to the antibiotic, and his mental state was improving. He did not seem restless or agitated when he was seen by our nurse about 15 minutes before he fell, so it is not clear why he tried to climb over the bed rail. There were two nurses in his bay, but one was attending to another patient at that time and the other had just left the bay to pick something from the nursing counter. He was therefore unfortunately briefly out of sight of both the nurses.'

She asks why you did not consider tying him to the bed, as he was at higher risk of falling.

Restraints should be used only if the individual is a threat to himself or others. The least-restrictive option should be chosen and used for the shortest possible time, as the use of restraints is not without risks. Patients who are restrained are at risk of worsening confusion or agitation, deep vein thrombosis, pressure ulcers, and deconditioning, so frequent re-evaluations are necessary.

Before tying a patient, it is preferable to first try less-restrictive forms of restraining, like using bed rails, 1:1 nursing, using a table tray in a geriatric chair, or chemical tranquilisation.

- Tell her that *physical restraint is only used as a last resort*.

    'We only do that in people who are agitated or restless and when we feel that they are at risk of harming themselves or others. Even in people who are agitated, we use it as a last-resort option and for the shortest possible time because it can sometimes make them more confused or agitated. Keeping them immobilised can also increase the risk of blood clots or bedsores.

    'Your father never displayed aggressive behaviour at any time, and his mental state was much better compared to how it was at the time of admission. Raising the side rail was also a form of restraint, and we least expected him to climb over it.'

She asks how he will be monitored, as it may not be so easy to spot a small change in the mental state or conscious level in a man like him who is already a bit confused.

- Tell her that *you will be monitoring his GCS*.

    'We will be monitoring him using a measure called the Glasgow Coma Scale. We'll regularly check his eyes, speech, and the movement of his limbs and give him a score ranging from 3 to 15. Right now, he is able to open his eyes on his own and move all his four limbs when we ask him to do so, but he is not completely aware of his surroundings, so we have given him a score of 14 out of 15. This was his baseline score even before he was admitted to the hospital.

    'If he is only able to open his eyes when we call him or apply some pressure on his body, or if he is not able to open his eyes at all, then the score for his eyes will be lowered accordingly. We have a similar grading system for how well he speaks or moves his limbs. If the overall score falls by two or more points, we'll repeat the brain scan to check if the blood clot is increasing in size. If the repeat scan shows that the blood clot is increasing in size, we'll inform the brain surgeon.'

She says she will be raising a complaint and seeking financial compensation for the harm that the hospital has caused.

Tell her that:

- *She is free to complain. It will not affect her father's medical care.*

'I am sorry that this is adding to your distress. I'll pass you the contact details of the patient liaison service office, to whom you can provide your feedback. I would like to assure you that making a complaint will not, in any way, affect how we care for your father.'

- *You will submit an incident report to ensure that any gaps are addressed.*

'We take the necessary steps to prevent people at high risk from falling, but unfortunately, this cannot be completely prevented. I'll submit an incident report, which will lead to a thorough investigation to look into what happened. We'll then be able to share more details of what went wrong. If we find any gaps, we'll certainly learn from them and put in measures in place to ensure that they are not repeated.'

If she has no further questions, end the conversation by telling her that her father should be back in the ward soon. You will continue to monitor him closely and inform the neurosurgeons promptly if there are any signs of deterioration. Tell her that the team will continue to update her on his progress.

SUMMARY

This scenario tests your skills in informing the daughter about an adverse event that her father has suffered. You will be expected to:

- Inform the daughter that her father fell from his bed, and sincerely apologise for what happened.
- Outline the steps that were taken soon after he fell and how you will continue to monitor him.
- Explain what precautions were taken to prevent him from falling, without sounding too defensive.
- Explain why he was not restrained.
- Tell her that she is free to make a complaint and this will not affect the care of her father.
- Tell her that an incident report will be submitted, and any gaps that are found will be addressed.

A variation of this case is disclosing a procedural complication to the daughter of an elderly man. He was admitted to the acute medical unit a little earlier with upper gastrointestinal bleeding. The decision was made to insert a central line through his right internal jugular vein, as he was haemodynamically unstable and peripheral venous access was difficult. There was no time to do the procedure under ultrasound guidance. You allowed your junior trainee doctor to first attempt the procedure, but he failed. Therefore, you took over and passed the line successfully.

After the procedure, the patient complained of shortness of breath. A bedside chest X-ray showed right-sided pneumothorax. As the pneumothorax was large and he was symptomatic, a chest drain was inserted, and he was commenced on high-flow oxygen. He was given three units of blood and commenced on intravenous proton pump inhibitor. The cause of his bleeding was not clear.

He has had no further bleeding since admission, and his blood pressure is stable at present. An endoscopy was planned this morning, but it has been deferred because of the pneumothorax and his high oxygen requirement. The daughter has just arrived, and she is yet to see her father.

You will be expected to:

- Tell her that her father was admitted with massive upper gastrointestinal bleeding, the cause of which is unclear.
- Tell her that he was haemodynamically unstable at the time of admission. He was given blood transfusion and commenced on intravenous proton pump inhibitor.
- Explain why the decision was taken to insert a central line.
- Tell her that the central line insertion has resulted in pneumothorax.
- Apologise to her and disclose that you allowed your junior trainee doctor to attempt the procedure.
- Explain how the pneumothorax is being managed and how long it will take for him to recover.
- Tell her that endoscopy has been deferred because of his high oxygen requirement, but he is stable at present, with no further bleeding.
- Tell her that you will file an incident report and learn from the mistake.

The 73-Year-Old Man Who Was Exposed to COVID in the Hospital

This 73-year-old man, with a background medical history of chronic obstructive pulmonary disease, ischaemic heart disease, diabetes mellitus, and bullous pemphigoid on long-term corticosteroid treatment, was admitted five days ago with fever and acute retention of urine. His white blood cell count and C-reactive protein were elevated. Urine culture grew *Escherichia coli*. Computed tomography of the abdomen and pelvis showed prostate enlargement. Prostate-specific antigen level and renal function were normal. He was commenced on amoxicillin–clavulanic acid at the time of admission with the intention to complete a seven-day course.

He has since clinically improved, and the catheter has been removed. The urologist has commenced him on finasteride and arranged to see him in his clinic in four weeks. The plan was to discharge him today, but the patient adjacent to him in the six-bedded bay tested positive for coronavirus disease 19 (COVID-19) yesterday, with a low cycle of transformation value. The COVID-positive patient was admitted for an unrelated problem on the same day as this man. He was swabbed, as he reported upper respiratory symptoms yesterday. He was shifted to a single room as soon as he was found to be COVID-positive. The other five patients in the bay have tested negative. The doctors and nurses who took care of these patients are well and asymptomatic.

The consultant feels that he can still be discharged with appropriate advice. He received his primary course of vaccination in 2021, followed by booster doses in 2022 and 2023. He is COVID-naïve. The patient has asked you to talk to his son, who has come to take him home.

- Introduce yourself, and check his identity and relationship to the patient. Ask what he has been told about his father so far.

He says he knows that his father was diagnosed with a urine infection and started on antibiotics. He hasn't been updated about the results of the scan and asks if it showed anything concerning.

- *Update him on the progress of his father.*

  'The scan shows that his prostate gland is enlarged. The prostate is a small gland that is located right below the bladder, which is the bag that stores urine. [Draw a diagram to

DOI: 10.1201/9781003533337-40

explain.] It surrounds the urethra, which is the passage that drains the urine from the bladder. Enlargement of the prostate is quite common in older men. An enlarged prostate can block the flow of urine through the urethra. It'll explain why he was not able to pee before he was admitted.

'We had to pass a tube to drain the urine. We have now removed it, as he is able to pee on his own. Anything that blocks the free flow of urine can increase the risk of infection, so we believe he developed the urine infection because of the prostate problem. He has responded well to the antibiotics, which he must continue taking for another two days to complete the course.

'We sought the advice of a urologist, who is a specialist on prostate problems. He has started him on a medication to improve the flow of urine and arranged to see him in his clinic in about four weeks.'

Pause and check his understanding. If he has no further questions, tell him that:

- *The patient in the adjacent bed tested positive for COVID.*

'Your father can be discharged today, but I must tell you about something that we discovered yesterday. The man in the bed adjacent to him tested positive for COVID. He was admitted on the same day as your father.'

The son gets upset when he hears that his father was exposed to someone with COVID in the ward. He asks why you did not keep his father isolated in the first place to avoid exposing him to infected people, as he is an elderly man with heart, lung, and skin problems.

- *His father has tested negative for COVID.*

'We shifted the patient with COVID to a single room as soon as tested positive. Your father has tested negative for COVID.'

- Explain that *there was no need to have isolated his father*.

'There is no need to isolate all elderly people or those with long-term medical conditions. We only isolate people who get admitted with an infection that they are likely to pass to the others, like COVID, tuberculosis, or chickenpox, or if the infection is caused by a bug that does not respond to the common antibiotics, because we don't want that bug to keep spreading. We also isolate people with very low blood counts because they are at risk of developing a serious illness when they catch an infection from the others.'

He asks why you did not test the patient in the adjacent bed much earlier. He is not happy that you allowed his father to lie next to him for four full days.

- Tell him that *there was no indication to test the COVID patient earlier*.

'The patient next to him only started coughing yesterday, which is why we tested him. He had no symptoms of COVID prior to that. We don't routinely test those who do not have any symptoms of COVID. It is likely that he caught the infection before he was

admitted to the hospital, as it can take a few days for a person to develop symptoms after catching the infection.'

The risk of transmission of COVID depends on (1) the duration of exposure, (2) proximity to the infected person, (3) whether the infected person was coughing, (4) whether one or both of them were wearing a mask, and (5) how well the area was ventilated. There is a higher risk of transmission if the duration of exposure was more than 15 minutes, the distance from the infected person was less than 1 m, the infected person was coughing, neither of them wore a mask, and the area where the exposure occurred was indoor and poorly ventilated. Being up to date with vaccination and recent COVID infection (in the last 90 days) may reduce the risk of infection.

Once the person gets COVID, factors that may increase the risk of progression to severe disease, hospitalisation, or death include (1) older age, (2) unvaccinated status or not being up to date with vaccination, and (3) having certain medical conditions (e.g. chronic obstructive pulmonary disease, liver cirrhosis, advanced chronic kidney disease, diabetes mellitus, cancer, immunosuppression due to disease or treatment). Anti-viral treatment (e.g. nirmatrelvir plus ritonavir or remdesivir) is recommended for patients with mild to moderate COVID who are at higher risk of progressing to severe disease.

He calms down after hearing your explanation. He asks after how many days they can be sure that he hasn't caught the infection and if he can be kept in the hospital until then.

- *Ask about his home situation.*

He tells you that his father lives with his mum about 2 miles away from where he lives. His mother is well, with no major medical problems, apart from wear and tear in her knees and a heart problem, for which she has a pacemaker. She still manages the cooking. They have employed a part-time cleaner to do the cleaning twice a week.

Tell him that:

- *His father can still be discharged.*

  'Your father may or may not have caught the infection. As he was at close distance to the man with COVID and neither of them wore a mask, his chance of getting COVID is indeed higher, but it is not 100%. If he has caught the infection, he is likely to develop the symptoms within the next week or so.

  'We don't have to keep him in the hospital until then. He can still be discharged home safely. Staying in the hospital for too long will only increase his risk of catching other kinds of infections that are more common in the hospital environment.'

- *He should monitor for symptoms of COVID.*

  'He should watch for symptoms of COVID, like fever, cough, sore throat, breathing difficulty, feeling tired, body aches, runny nose, and loss of taste or smell. The symptoms are very similar to those of flu.'

The son says he developed COVID twice and knows what the symptoms are. He asks if he should bring his father to the hospital if he develops these symptoms.

Tell him that:

- *If he develops symptoms, he should do a lateral flow test* (antigen rapid test).

  'If he develops symptoms, he should test himself using the kit that we provide. If the test is negative, he should keep testing every day for three consecutive days. Our nurse will teach him how to do this himself. There is no need to do the test if he doesn't develop any symptoms. The purpose of testing him is to decide if he needs to be started on treatment.'

- *If the lateral flow test is positive, he should contact his GP so that he can be started on anti-viral treatment.*

  'If he tests positive for COVID, he should get in touch with his GP, who will suggest treatments to reduce the risk of the infection becoming severe. The treatment can be given in the form of tablets or as a drip in the hospital. The doctor will decide which treatment is best for him. These treatments are only prescribed for people with certain long-term medical conditions.
  'Most people who catch COVID have mild symptoms and get better within a few days. Not everyone needs admission to a hospital.'

- *He should isolate himself if he develops symptoms.*

  'If he develops symptoms, he should stay at home and isolate himself, even if the test result is negative. He should avoid contact with people for five days, starting from the day he takes the test. This should be extended to ten days for people with weak immunity, as they are at risk of getting seriously ill if they catch COVID. If he doesn't develop any symptoms, there is no need for him to be confined at home.'

End the conversation by summarising the main points. Tell him that you will give him an information sheet on COVID. He should (1) monitor his symptoms, (2) do a lateral flow test when he develops symptoms, and (3) start anti-viral treatment as soon as possible if the result is positive.

SUMMARY

This scenario tests your skills in talking to a son about his father, who was inadvertently exposed to COVID-19 in the hospital. You will be expected to:

- Update the son on the progress of his father.
- Tell him that his father was exposed to COVID-19 in the hospital but he can still be discharged.
- Reassure him that most people with COVID-19 recover within a few days.
- Explore his situation at home and social support.

- Talk convincingly and explain clearly that (1) he should monitor for symptoms, (2) do a lateral flow test if he becomes symptomatic, and (3) contact his GP to start anti-viral treatment if the result is positive.
- Provide advice on some general measures to follow.

A variation of this case is talking to a pregnant woman in her first trimester who was admitted to the hospital a couple of days ago with acute exacerbation of her asthma. Her symptoms have markedly improved with prednisolone and nebulised bronchodilators, and the plan was to discharge her today. However, you just found out that the elderly woman in her adjacent bed in the six-bedded bay developed ophthalmic shingles yesterday. She was transferred to a single room straightaway. The swab from the vesicle was later reported as positive for herpes zoster virus.

According to the infection control team, the exposure of the pregnant woman could be considered significant, taking into account the duration of exposure, the distance between them, and the presence of vesicles over an exposed part of the body. She has never had chickenpox and not received the varicella vaccine. The consultant in infectious diseases has therefore suggested checking her varicella zoster virus IgG and giving her acyclovir from day 7–14 of exposure if the result is negative. The intent of giving acyclovir is to reduce the risk of varicella pneumonia and fetal varicella syndrome.

You will be expected to tell her that:

- The patient in her adjacent bed has tested positive for herpes zoster.
- The infection control team felt that her exposure was significant.

Note: The exposure is considered significant if the person was exposed to (1) someone with chickenpox, (2) disseminated shingles, (3) an immunocompetent patient with shingles in an exposed area, or (4) an immunosuppressed patient with shingles in any part of the body.

- You would like to check her varicella zoster virus IgG, as she has never had chickenpox or received the varicella vaccine.
- If the varicella zoster virus IgG is positive, no further action is needed.
- If the result is negative, she is at risk of getting chickenpox. There is a higher risk of severe chickenpox and fetal varicella syndrome (more likely if exposed during the first 20 weeks of pregnancy).

Note: Fetal varicella syndrome manifests as microcephaly, cataracts, limb hypoplasia, and growth retardation.

- The consultant in infectious diseases has recommended acyclovir to be taken for eight days from day 7–14 from exposure. Acyclovir will not prevent chickenpox, but it will significantly reduce the severity of the disease and the risk of fetal varicella syndrome. It is safe during pregnancy. Common side effects include headache, dizziness, nausea, vomiting, and diarrhoea.

Note: There is a severe shortage of varicella zoster immunoglobulin (VZ Ig) in the UK, and moreover, it has sub-optimal efficacy in pregnant women, hence the recommendation to use acyclovir. VZ Ig is only used in those with severe hyperemesis, gastrointestinal malabsorption, or renal impairment under expert guidance.

You should manage her emotions appropriately after you break the news of her exposure to shingles (e.g. anger, anxiety, distress, fear).

Case 36

The 27-Year-Old Woman with a Severe Allergic Reaction to Sulfasalazine

This 27-year-old lady was diagnosed with seropositive rheumatoid arthritis (RA) and commenced on sulfasalazine about three weeks ago. She was also given an intramuscular injection of depot corticosteroid at that time for symptom relief. Her rheumatologist wanted to start her on methotrexate but instead chose sulfasalazine, as she told her that she would like to try for a second child once her arthritis was controlled. She was in good health prior to being diagnosed with RA.

She has presented to the acute medical unit (AMU) this morning with a two-day history of widespread erythematous rash and severe oral mucositis. She just increased the dose of sulfasalazine to three tablets a day this week as advised by her rheumatologist. She reported that she did not take any other medication, including those that can be bought over the counter. She has no known allergies. She was diagnosed with toxic epidermal necrolysis, most likely secondary to sulfasalazine.

Her vital signs have been normal since admission, with no evidence of internal organ involvement. Her blood counts, liver function tests, serum albumin, renal function, blood glucose, venous bicarbonate, and chest X-ray are all normal. You are the medical registrar in the AMU. You have the patient's permission to talk to her husband, who is waiting to find out what the problem is.

Stevens–Johnson syndrome (SJS) and toxic epidermal necrolysis (TEN) are characterised by acute skin rash, mucous membrane involvement, blisters, and skin desquamation. It is called SJS when <10% of the body surface area is involved, SJS–TEN overlap when 10–30% is involved, and TEN when >30% is involved. Both SJS and TEN are caused by a drug reaction. The usual culprits are allopurinol, sulfasalazine, penicillin, non-steroidal anti-inflammatory drugs, and anti-convulsant drugs.

The skin plays an important role in (1) preventing percutaneous loss of fluid, electrolytes, and proteins; (2) forming a physical barrier to prevent invasion by microorganisms; and (3) maintaining core body temperature. Hence, patients with loss of skin function due to extensive involvement by a disease process are prone to developing fluid and electrolyte disturbances, protein–energy malnutrition, infections, and hypothermia. TEN is associated with high mortality.

Management of TEN may include (1) fluid resuscitation for those with hypotension, (2) correction of electrolyte disturbances, (3) broad-spectrum antibiotics for those with evidence of infection, (4) opioids for pain relief, (5) topical treatment with a bland emollient to reduce the discomfort and form a protective barrier, (6) antiseptic mouthwash, (7) nasogastric tube feeding for those with reduced oral intake due to severe oral mucosal involvement, and (8) maintenance of room temperature between 30 and 32°C. Those with upper airway mucosal involvement are at risk of respiratory compromise and may require intubation, while those with eye involvement are at risk of blindness due to keratitis, corneal ulceration, and scarring.

- Introduce yourself, and check his identity and relationship to the patient. Tell him that you have come to talk to him about his wife. Start by obtaining a brief history.

He says his wife had been complaining of pain and swelling in her hands and feet for quite a while. She saw a rheumatologist, who diagnosed rheumatoid arthritis and commenced her on sulfasalazine three weeks ago. She gradually increased the dosage according to her advice and went up to three tablets a day this week.

Her joint pains were much better after the steroid injection, and she was fine until two days ago, when she started complaining of itching. She stopped taking sulfasalazine straightaway. The rash appeared on the following day, and it gradually progressed over the next several hours to involve almost the entire body and her mouth. He wants to know what the problem is and if it is related to the sulfasalazine.

Tell him that:

- *She has developed a severe allergic reaction, most likely due to sulfasalazine.*

'Yes, we suspect she has developed a severe allergic reaction to the sulfasalazine. Our immune system is only meant to attack anything that is harmful, like bacteria or viruses. Allergy *simply means that the immune system also reacts to harmless particles, like medications, dust, peanuts, or seafood. It can manifest in different ways.*
'The type of allergic reaction that she has developed leads to the formation of blisters, peeling of the skin, and inflammation of the mouth and eyes. We call this toxic epidermal necrolysis. [Write down on a piece of paper.] Toxic because it is related to a toxin or medication, epidermis is the superficial layer of the skin, and necrolysis is the medical term for peeling of the skin. Sulfasalazine is known to cause this kind of reaction in a small number of people who take it. We think sulfasalazine is the most likely culprit because she hasn't been taking any other medication.'*

He becomes quite concerned when he hears that this is a severe allergic reaction. He asks what they should expect in the coming days and how long it will take for her to get well.

After saying a few comforting words, tell him that:

- *It is difficult to predict how long it will take for her to recover.*

'At this stage, it is difficult to predict how long it'll take for her to recover. It could possibly take several weeks.'*

- *She will be closely monitored.*

  '*I'm afraid the skin rash may continue to worsen. A severe allergic reaction can also potentially harm the internal organs, like the lungs, liver, and kidneys. We'll continue to monitor her closely. Right now, her temperature, pulse, breathing, and blood pressure are normal, and there is nothing to suggest that any of her internal organs are affected. Her chest X-ray, blood counts, liver and kidney tests, and glucose are all normal.*'

- *You will be seeking the opinion of a dermatologist.*

  '*We'll be asking a skin specialist to provide expert advice on the treatment of her condition.*'

He asks how she will be managed and if there are any treatments that can help heal the skin faster.

Tell him that:

- *There are no medications that have been shown to modify the course of TEN.*

  '*There are no medications that can help heal the skin faster. The skin will gradually heal on its own.*'

- *Extensive skin inflammation could lead to fluid and electrolyte imbalance, increased risk of infection, and hypothermia.*

  '*The skin helps prevent the loss of fluids and salts from the body, provide a barrier to stop bacteria from getting in, and maintain our body temperature by reducing the loss of heat. An extensive inflammation of the skin could therefore lead to loss of fluids and salts from the body, higher risk of infection, and lowering of the body temperature. We'll give her a drip and make sure she gets enough fluids and salts, start her on an antibiotic if she develops any signs of infection, and place her in a room with an ideal temperature.*'

- *You will appropriately manage her symptoms until she recovers.*

  '*We'll regularly apply a moisturiser over her skin. It'll not only provide comfort but also reduce the loss of fluids and heat from the body. We'll use an antiseptic mouthwash to reduce her risk of getting an infection in the mouth. Once the skin peels off, the raw areas of the skin can cause pain. We'll give her a painkiller if she complains of any pain. She won't be able to eat for quite some time, so we may have to consider temporarily feeding her through a tube inserted via the nose and placed in the stomach. We'll keep you updated on a daily basis to let you know how she is progressing.*'

He asks why this happened to her and if it could have been predicted earlier.

Tell him that:

- *The allergic reaction could not have been predicted beforehand.*

  '*We do not know why some people react like this to certain medications. For some medications, we can predict the risk of developing an adverse reaction by doing a blood test, but it is not possible to do that for sulfasalazine.*'

- *She must avoid taking sulfasalazine or similar drugs in the future.*

  '*She should avoid taking sulfasalazine and another medication called Bactrim, which is used to treat urine infections. She can take all the other medications. We will record this allergy in her medical notes so that everyone is aware. Once she recovers, I am sure her rheumatologist will consider an alternative medication to control her arthritis.*'

He asks if you think he should make a complaint against the rheumatologist.

- Find out what he is unhappy about. *Ask if they were told about the risk of allergy* before sulfasalazine was commenced.

He says they were told about the risk of allergy but that it was very rare. She agreed to take the pill because she was told that the benefits outweighed the risks. She wouldn't have agreed if she had known that she was going to react like this.

- Tell him that *there are no grounds to complain* (the tone in which this is said is important).

  '*Her rheumatologist prescribed the sulfasalazine with the intention of improving her arthritis. This kind of reaction is very rare, indeed. It couldn't have been predicted beforehand. Please do not feel that this has happened because of a medical error. It can happen to anyone. It is very unfortunate that she had this reaction. Let's focus on what happens from now on and hope that she gets well soon.*'

End the conversation by telling him that the medical team will continue to update them regularly. The dermatologist and rheumatologist will see her shortly. You will be happy to come back and talk to him if he has any further questions.

There are three parts in a doctor–patient interaction: (1) making a diagnosis, (2) giving advice, and (3) providing treatment. The Bolam–Bolitho test, which is used in civil courts to determine if a doctor was negligent, only applies to diagnosis and treatment. Under the Bolam–Bolitho test, a doctor cannot be considered negligent if they are deemed to have acted in accordance with a responsible body of medical opinion (i.e. if their peers would have acted similarly if they had been in the same situation), *provided the court finds the opinion of the peers to be logical.*

The Montgomery test is used to determine if the doctor was negligent in providing advice. It involves asking the following three questions:

1. Was relevant information not communicated to the patient?

2. If not, was the doctor in possession of that information?
3. If yes, was the doctor justified in withholding that information from the patient?

For example, a doctor may be justified in withholding information about the risks and proceeding with emergency treatment of a person without capacity.

In this case, had the rheumatologist not communicated the risk of allergy before commencing sulfasalazine, she would have breached her duty of care, as she was in possession of that information and there was no justification to withhold it.

SUMMARY

This scenario tests your skills in talking to the husband about a medication-related severe adverse effect that his wife was already warned about. You will be expected to:

- Explain to the husband that his wife has had a severe allergic reaction to sulfasalazine.
- Outline the management of TEN.
- Warn him that the skin rash could worsen and there is a potential risk of internal organ involvement.
- Tell him that this reaction could not have been predicted beforehand.
- Tell him that she must avoid taking sulfasalazine and similar drugs, like cotrimoxazole, in the future.
- Gently point out that there are no grounds to complain against the rheumatologist.

A variation of this case is talking to the wife of a 63-year-old man who was admitted to a hospital a few days ago with unstable angina. His coronary angiogram showed significant stenosis of the right coronary and left anterior descending artery. Angioplasty was performed, with placement of stents in both the blood vessels. He was commenced on dual anti-platelet therapy (DAPT) with aspirin and clopidogrel and advised to take them for six months before switching to single anti-platelet therapy.

Three days after commencing DAPT, he developed massive rectal bleeding, leading to haemodynamic instability. He was fluid-resuscitated and given blood transfusion. Both anti-platelet drugs were withheld. As the computed tomographic mesenteric angiogram showed evidence of active haemorrhage, interventional radiology-guided angioembolisation was performed. According to the gastroenterologist, his bleeding was most likely due to diverticular disease. The wife is unhappy and blames the anti-platelet therapy for his bleeding.

You will be expected to:

- Find out what her concerns are.
- Explain how his unstable angina was managed and why he had to be commenced on anti-platelet therapy.
- Explain how his gastrointestinal bleeding was managed.

- Tell her that the bleeding was most likely due to diverticular disease and may have been aggravated by anti-platelet therapy.
- Ask if they were told about the risk of bleeding with anti-platelet therapy.
- Reassure her that anti-platelet therapy will soon be resumed in consultation with the cardiologist and gastroenterologist, as their benefits outweigh the risks.

The 69-Year-Old Woman Whose Cord Compression Was Not Diagnosed in Time

This 69-year-old woman, with a background history of diabetes mellitus, hyperlipidaemia, and renal calculi, was admitted to the acute medical unit (AMU) last night with a one-day history of low back pain and urinary retention. She denied fever or constitutional symptoms. Her husband reported that she had been 'off legs'.

Her vital signs were satisfactory. She was seen by the junior doctor, who recorded 'renal angle tenderness' and a 'distended bladder'. Her post-void residual urine volume was about 400 mL. Investigations arranged by him showed normal full blood count, liver function tests, and serum creatinine. There were 64 white blood cells and 12 red blood cells in her urine. He diagnosed pyelonephritis and commenced her on ceftriaxone and paracetamol.

The consultant who examined her this morning noted that the power in both her legs was grade 2/5, sensory perception was diminished throughout both her lower limbs, and plantar response was extensor bilaterally. An urgent magnetic resonance imaging (MRI) scan of the spine showed a mass at the level of T10/T11 compressing the spinal cord, which was possibly an epidural abscess.

The orthopaedic surgeon has taken her to the theatre for urgent operative decompression and biopsy of the mass. He felt that her prognosis for recovery of leg function was poor because of the delayed referral. Unfortunately, there was no record of a neurological examination of her legs on the previous night. You were the registrar in the AMU last night. Your task is to talk to the distraught junior doctor. He is deeply upset that he missed the spinal cord compression.

The term 'second victim' refers to a healthcare worker who becomes traumatised as a result of being involved in a medical error. The healthcare worker may experience shame, guilt, anxiety, depression, post-traumatic stress, problems sleeping, difficulty in concentrating at work, a loss of confidence, and burnout. In extreme cases, they may entertain thoughts of quitting the profession or committing suicide.

Medical errors are seldom caused by the fault of a single person. They are often due to a combination of human and system factors (e.g. staffing issues, hectic working environment, inadequate training). There should be a 'just culture' (looking at both human and system factors) and a support system in place to enable second victims to *thrive* and not just *survive*

DOI: 10.1201/9781003533337-42

(become isolated or suffer in silence) or *drop out*. There will be more negative consequences if the healthcare worker is not supported well.

There is no need for you to introduce yourself or confirm his identity, as you worked with him last night. Pretend that you know him well! In real life, you should take him to a private place to chat.

- Start by asking how he is feeling. Do not ask him to narrate what happened ('*How are you feeling?*' not '*Tell me what happened*').

He says he feels distraught. He is deeply upset that the patient won't be able to walk again because of his mistake. He becomes emotional and laments that he is not fit to be in this profession anymore.

- *Provide emotional first aid.*

  '*I understand. It is natural to feel upset and dejected. We all make mistakes. I've made a lot of mistakes too. We are only human. No one is perfect. However, when a mistake is made in healthcare, it is seldom the fault of a single person. There will be an investigation to find out why things went wrong. We all want to support you so that you get over this and come out stronger.*'

While providing emotional first aid, do not give false reassurances, like 'Don't worry, you will be fine', just to soothe the person. We do not know for sure if she had similar neurological findings at the time of presentation or they only progressed through the night. Nonetheless, it is clear that he must have (1) at least performed a basic neurological examination, as she was 'off her legs' and had urinary retention, and (2) asked either you or the orthopaedic registrar to see her. After an incident report is submitted, the investigators will also look at the system factors that led to this error ('What led to this mistake?' and not just 'Who made this mistake?').

He continues to talk. He says he is not trying to offer excuses but it was a busy night and the phone was constantly ringing. He was distracted by numerous other tasks. On top of that, he was tired and exhausted, as he did not manage to sleep well yesterday. He did not ask you to review this patient as it seemed like a straightforward urinary tract infection to him. He was swayed by the history of renal calculi and thought the back pain and paraspinal tenderness pointed to pyelonephritis. He did not make much of the urinary retention, which also seemed to point to a urinary tract infection in a lady of her age. He was taught as a medical student that it is common for elderly people to go 'off legs' when they get an infection. It just slipped his mind to perform a neurological examination of her legs.

- *Sympathise and offer your support.*

  '*I thought so. I know it was quite busy last night. No one comes to work with the intention to harm people, and we cannot avoid such mistakes altogether, no matter how careful we are. The important thing is to learn from this incident and make sure it does not happen again.*'

- Tell him *what symptoms he might experience in the coming days to weeks and about the avenues of support that are available.*

'It'll take some time for you to get over this. This might affect your mood, make you feel guilty, disturb your sleep at night, and make it difficult for you to concentrate at work. It is only natural for any of us to experience such emotions when something like this happens.

'If you need to take some time off work, please let the roster planners and your supervisor know. We have peers who are experts on providing counselling to our healthcare workers who are distressed. We can ask them to talk to you. I am sure you'll find that immensely helpful.'

He asks what will happen next and if the patient and her family members will be told about the mistake.

Tell him that:

- **A full investigation will be conducted.**

'An incident report will be submitted. A full investigation will be conducted to find out what went wrong – just like how the black box is studied carefully after a plane crash. The findings of the investigations will help us look at the gaps and make sure the mistakes are not repeated.'

- Tell him that *an open and honest disclosure will be made to her once the investigations are completed.*

'We have a duty of candour. It is important to be open and honest, so she must be told about the delay in referral. Whether an earlier referral would have changed her outcome is a different matter altogether. It is possible that she was already very weak last night, in which case an earlier operation may not have changed the outcome significantly. It's too early to speculate. We will know only after obtaining a more detailed history from her or her family members about the time course of events and seeking opinions from different consultants.'

He asks if you think they will sue him if the internal investigations conclude that an earlier referral would have changed her outcome.

- Tell him that *he should let his medical defence organisation know.*

'If the consensus opinion is that an earlier referral would have changed her outcome and we tell her that, she might complain or even forgive us – we don't know. When we have that conversation, we will apologise to her, honestly tell her what went wrong, and assure her that we will learn from this mistake. Those are the three things that patients generally expect from us. There may be a discussion on financial compensation as well. I would suggest that you let your medical defence organisation know. They are experts in dealing with medicolegal complaints, and they'll guide you.'

Dealing with medical error is not part of the medical school curriculum, so most junior doctors may not be fully aware of what happens when a complaint is made by a patient. The process for dealing with complaints may vary in different parts of the world. Most complaints are a result of poor communication, which are usually resolved locally. Only a small proportion of complaints are of a more serious nature and are caused by negligence, resulting in patient harm.

Depending on the extent of harm or level of satisfaction with the initial response from the hospital, the complainant may decide to escalate the complaint to the medical council or file a lawsuit. Possible outcomes may include (1) no action against the healthcare worker (if no evidence of negligence is found), (2) 'out-of-court' settlement, or (3) financial compensation as ordered by the civil court. Additionally, depending on the nature of the error, disciplinary action may be taken against the doctor either by the organisation or the medical council, but this is not common. It is good to inform the medical defence organisation early so that they can be well prepared and assist the person(s) against whom the complaint is made.

It is advisable to discuss her case in a morbidity meeting so that the learning points can be shared with the others, but this need not be mentioned to him at this stage. The thought that he will be 'named and shamed' is likely to make him more anxious, although that is not the intent of the presentation.

He asks if this incident will affect his training opportunities. He is keen to apply for specialty training after passing the MRCP.

- Tell him that *his overall performance will be taken into account*.

  'Let's not think that far. Whether or not you are able to get into specialty training will depend on your overall record. I don't think it'll be affected by this one incident. I am sure the program directors will be aware that a majority of medical errors are committed by competent people working in a complex healthcare system fraught with system factors that are bound to fail from time to time.'

End the conversation by asking him to go home and rest. Tell him that he will be asked to provide his account of the events, but reassure him that he will be provided with the necessary support. It is too early to jump to any conclusions, as it depends on how well she recovers after the operation and the outcome of the investigations. Regardless of whether the outcome would have been different had an earlier referral been made, it is a good idea to alert the medical defence organisation. Ask him to look out for you if he wants to talk about this further.

SUMMARY

This scenario tests your skills in talking to a distraught junior doctor who has committed a medical error. You will be expected to:

- Ask how he is feeling, and listen to his side of the story.
- Provide emotional first aid.

- Tell him about the avenues of support that are available.
- Tell him that an open and honest disclosure will be made to the patient but only after the investigations have concluded.
- Advise him to let his medical defence organisation know.
- Address his anxieties regarding future training opportunities, his career, and potential lawsuit.

A variation of this case is talking to a junior doctor who is reported to have performance issues (although this is usually done by the educational or clinical supervisor). You should (1) start the conversation by asking the trainee how he is getting on, (2) focus on the positive aspects of his work, (3) tell him about the poor feedback and source of feedback, (4) hear his side of the story, (5) determine what the problem is (knowledge and skills, professionalism, or health-related), and (6) provide constructive feedback and give him a performance improvement plan with targets to be achieved within a certain time frame.

The solution will depend on what the problem is. If the trainee has competency issues, for example, some possible solutions may be closer supervision, shadowing a more experienced junior doctor, placing the trainee with supportive or nurturing consultants, temporarily taking him off night calls, or looking at ways of improving his working environment. You should refer the matter to his educational supervisor, who will have an elaborate discussion with him and document it in his record.

Section VI

End-of-Life Issues

The 69-Year-Old Woman Who Wants to Make a Living Will

This 69-year-old lady has multiple medical problems, including hypertension, diabetes mellitus, hyperlipidaemia, chronic kidney disease stage 3, and heart failure with reduced ejection fraction. She has been admitted to the hospital thrice in the last 12 months with fluid overload.

She wants to make a living will and wishes to discuss it with you.

- After the initial introduction, start with an open-ended question and *ask how you can help.*

She says she heard from a friend that she can make a living will if she does not wish to receive certain treatments in the future. Her sister, who died from COVID four years ago, suffered for several weeks when she was connected to a breathing machine. She herself has been admitted three times in the last year with breathing problems and is worried that she, too, may be connected to a machine one day. She doesn't want to experience what her sister went through and would like to go peacefully when the time comes. She wants your advice before making this will.

The legal term for a living will is *advance decision to refuse treatment* (ADRT). It can be done by any adult ($\geq$18 years of age in the UK) with mental capacity. It lets them state in advance any treatments (e.g. cardiopulmonary resuscitation, mechanical ventilation, artificial feeding) that they do not wish to receive should they lose their mental capacity in the future. This is in line with the Mental Capacity Act 2005, which aims to empower vulnerable people by enabling them to plan ahead and express their wishes and preferences.

The person, however, cannot refuse basic care (e.g. feeding, hydration, hygiene), ask for euthanasia, or demand treatments that are not clinically indicated. Additionally, those who are detained under the Mental Health Act cannot refuse treatment for their mental health condition (with the exception of electroconvulsive therapy). An ADRT can be made verbally or in writing. If life-sustaining treatments are refused, the ADRT *must* be made in writing and specifically state that the refusal applies even if it is likely to lead to death. The document should be signed and dated in the presence of a witness.

DOI: 10.1201/9781003533337-44

An ADRT is legally binding in the UK provided it is *valid* and *applicable*. For an ADRT to be valid, it must be made by a person with capacity (it will take effect only after they lose capacity). It should be done voluntarily without coercion, and the person should have been provided with enough information about the implications of refusing the treatment. For the ADRT to be applicable, the person should state not only the treatment that is being refused but also the circumstances in which the refusal should apply ('I do not wish to be connected to a breathing machine if I get admitted to the hospital with pneumonia or fluid in my lungs even if it is likely to lead to death').

After expressing your sadness for the death of her sister, you should:

- *Ask about her family.*

Are those who are close to her (e.g. spouse, children, siblings) aware of her wishes?

She is retired and lives with her husband. Her elder son lives in Scotland, and the younger in Australia. All three are aware that she does not want aggressive interventions. Her husband and elder son are in agreement with her wishes, but the younger son feels that she should not refuse life-saving treatments.

- *Make sure she understands the implications of refusing treatments*, especially those that are life-sustaining.

'I fully appreciate why you do not wish to be connected to a breathing machine, but not everyone remains on it for weeks. It depends. Some people only need the machine for a few days. The doctors may decide to connect you to a breathing machine if there is excess fluid in the lungs that cannot be removed with medicines or you develop a bad lung infection. Do you realise that in such a situation, your life could be at risk if you are not connected to the breathing machine?'

She says she understands that she may need the support of a breathing machine if she develops fluid collection in the lungs or a bad lung infection. She also understands that she may not need the machine for more than a few days and it could be life-saving. She does not wish to go through that suffering.

She clearly has capacity as (1) there is no impairment of her mind or brain and (2) she is able to comprehend, retain the information, weigh the pros and cons, and communicate her decision. The informed decision of a person with capacity cannot be overridden even if it is irrational.

- *Explain what an ADRT is and how she should prepare one.*

'Once you have thought through this carefully and decided what sort of treatments you do not wish to receive, I would suggest that you write them down. You should sign and date this document in the presence of a witness – the witness should sign it as well. We call this an advance decision to refuse treatment. In case you lose the ability to express your wishes in the future, we are legally obliged to comply with what you have put down in the advance decision.'

- *Guide her on some important dos and don'ts.*

'There are a few dos and don'ts to remember while preparing this document. You can only use this document to refuse, not ask for a particular treatment, as that will be decided by the doctors. You cannot refuse basic care, like food and water, or ask for your life to be ended. If you are refusing a life-sustaining treatment, you should specifically state in the document that you understand that your life will be at risk if you refuse that treatment. In an emergency, if it is not clear whether your refusal applies to that particular situation, the doctors will go ahead and give you the treatment that you refuse, so it is important to be as specific as possible. If you change your mind in the future, you can always modify the document or even cancel it completely.'

- Tell her that *she should make her healthcare team and family members aware of the ADRT.*

'I would suggest that you give copies of this document to your GP and hospital consultant so that they can file it in your notes. It is also a good idea to give a copy to your family members or close friends, so that they, too, are aware.'

- *Ask her to think through the other invasive treatments that she does not wish to receive.*

'There are other treatments that involve performing procedures like resuscitation, dialysis, and insertion of feeding tubes. If the heart stops beating, we perform resuscitation, which involves pressing the chest, delivering shocks, and giving medicines to restart the heart. Those in whom resuscitation is successful may be connected to a breathing machine. If your kidney function declines, you may be connected to a machine to remove the wastes from your body. If you are unable to swallow, we may pass a tube into your stomach to feed you. Think about those as well. Take your time.'

Pause for a while, and invite any questions before proceeding further.

- Tell her that *she can additionally set up a lasting power of attorney* (LPA).

'You can also set up something called a lasting power of attorney. It is a legal document that will allow someone you trust to make decisions on your behalf after you lose the ability to make decisions yourself. The trusted person you appoint will act as your attorney. Based on what you have told me, your elder son may be more suited to be your attorney if you decide to do this. You can appoint an attorney not only for health but also to manage your financial matters.'

An ordinary power of attorney can be made for financial decisions. It is valid only until the person has mental capacity, whereas an LPA will become valid *after* the person loses capacity. If the person has done both an ADRT and an LPA, whichever was made more recently will take priority. For example, if person creates an LPA *after* the ADRT and the attorney is given the authority in respect of a certain decision, consent should be sought from the attorney before administering the treatment in question. The attorney can refuse the treatment only if it is in the best interests of the person.

She asks how she will be managed in case she doesn't get around to making an ADRT or LPA and loses her mental capacity in the future.

- Tell her that *the healthcare team will then act in her best interests*.

  'We'll then act in your best interests, which simply means that we will make decisions based on your wishes and preferences and choose the treatment that we think will give you the best possible outcome. We'll have to ask your family members about your wishes and preferences, and it is not always easy.'

- If there is a conflict between family members, they can approach the court to appoint a proxy decision-maker, also known as a court-appointed deputy.

  'Another option is for your family members to approach the court to appoint someone as a deputy to act on your behalf if they are not able to agree on how you should be treated, but it is an expensive, complicated, and time-consuming process.'

Note: Donee is the attorney named in the LPA by the person, and *deputy* is the person appointed by the court. If it appears that the donee or deputy is not acting in the best interests of the person who has lost capacity, it can be brought to the attention of the court of protection.

She asks if she is allowed to put down what she prefers so that you know what her likes and dislikes are if and when she loses her awareness.

- *Tell her about advance statement.*

  'You can prepare another document called an advance statement, in which you can pretty much say anything, like what foods you like, whether you prefer a bath or shower, what music you like, where you would like to die, and so on. It is not legally binding like an advance decision or the lasting power of attorney, but the healthcare team will try to follow what you put down in the advance statement.'

End the discussion by briefly summarising the main points about an ADRT, LPA, and advance statement. Tell her that you will give her some information about useful websites that she can refer to. Tell her that she can take her time and you will be happy to see her again if she needs further advice.

SUMMARY

This scenario tests your skills in guiding someone who wishes to prepare a living will. You will be expected to:

- Find out why she wishes to make a living will.
- Assess her mental capacity.
- Make sure she understands the implications of refusing treatments, especially those that are life-sustaining.

- Provide an overview of how to prepare an ADRT.
- Tell her about (1) lasting power of attorney, (2) the difference between an ADRT and an advance statement, and (3) court-appointed deputy.
- Tell her that the medical team will act in her best interests if she does not prepare an ADRT or LPA and loses her mental capacity in the future.

The 82-Year-Old Woman for Whom the Medical Team Feels That CPR Should Not Be Attempted

This 82-year-old woman has multiple medical problems, including advanced dementia, ischaemic heart disease, heart failure with reduced ejection fraction, hypertension, diabetes mellitus, and chronic kidney disease (CKD) stage 4. She was admitted four days ago with breathlessness, which was attributed to heart failure and progression of her CKD.

She has clinically improved after fluid restriction and intravenous diuretics. She has been weaned off oxygen and switched back to oral furosemide. Her vital signs are satisfactory, and the plan is to discharge her soon.

The medical team feels that in the event of a cardiac arrest, cardiopulmonary resuscitation (CPR) should not be attempted in view of her multiple medical problems. Your task is to discuss her resuscitation status with the daughter. The patient herself has no mental capacity.

- Introduce yourself, and confirm the identity of the daughter and her relationship to the patient. Find out what she has been told already.

She says she is relieved to see that her mother is so much better since coming to the hospital. She asks if you could optimise her medications, as she keeps getting admitted with breathing trouble and this is already her third admission this year.

Tell her that:

- *She has been treated with fluid restriction and diuretics.*

'She is indeed much better compared to how she was four days ago. She keeps getting breathless because of her heart and kidney problems. Her heart is weak, which is causing fluid to collect in the lungs. As her kidneys are not working well, it is making it difficult for her to get rid of the excess fluid from the body.

'We gave her a medicine through the vein to remove the excess fluid from her body and strictly restricted the amount of fluid that she can drink in a day. She also needed some oxygen for a few days. She has responded well to these treatments. Her heartbeat, breathing, blood pressure, and oxygen level in her blood are all back to normal. We are hoping to discharge her in a day or two.'

DOI: 10.1201/9781003533337-45

- *There is no cure for her heart failure and chronic kidney disease. She is likely to gradually deteriorate despite the medical treatments.*

'*By restricting the amount of fluid that she drinks and giving the water tablet to stop the build-up of excess fluid in her body, we can try to improve her breathing and reduce the chance of further admissions, but this cannot be avoided completely. I am afraid there is no cure for her heart and kidney problems. Despite our best efforts, these problems are likely to gradually worsen with time.*'

- *Cardiac arrest is an eventual possibility. You would like to discuss with her the course of action to take when she arrests.*

'*I am sorry to be blunt, but a time will come when her heart will stop. We call this cardiac arrest. It can happen at home or when she is in the hospital. I would like to discuss with you what we think we should do when that happens, rather than leaving it to the last minute. It is good to have a clear plan now, as we obviously cannot be discussing that after her heart stops.*'

It is important to phrase it as 'what we think we should do', as you are conveying the decision of the medical team and not asking for her consent to not resuscitate her mother. Families may oppose your decision and ask you to 'do everything possible', but if the medical team feels that the patient is unlikely to benefit from resuscitation, it should be conveyed gently and empathetically.

- *Ask if her mother has ever expressed her wishes* about how she would like to be treated if she became very unwell.

'*Has she ever expressed her wishes verbally or in writing about how she would like to be treated in case she became very unwell?*'

Note: Patients can only express their wishes to decline. They cannot demand treatments that are not clinically indicated or appropriate. In case she expressed her wishes to be resuscitated no matter what, the medical team is not obliged to comply.

She says she understands what you are saying but she hasn't thought that far. She agrees that it is better to be prepared for that eventuality. Her mother has never openly discussed how she would like to be treated in the final days of her life, so she is not sure what she would have preferred.

You should now explain the process of resuscitation and tell her why the medical team feels that she should not be resuscitated in the event of a cardiac arrest. Note that if the patient had had capacity, this discussion should have taken place with her directly.

- First, *check her understanding of CPR.*

'*Have you heard of resuscitation? What do you know about that?*'

She says she knows that it is a process of bringing someone back to life when the heart stops. She has seen this on TV dramas.

- *Explain what CPR involves.*

'Yes, correct. It involves pressing the chest up and down, giving shocks, giving medicines to restart the heart, and passing a tube down the throat to connect to a breathing machine. We call this CPR.'

- Tell her that **CPR is not universally successful and it is not ideal for everyone.**

'We don't do CPR for everyone. For some people, we decide in advance to not try to restart the heart. Contrary to what you see on TV dramas, CPR is not successful in most people.

'Even if it is successful, some people end up having a poor quality of life after that because of the brain damage that occurs during the time when the heart stops. Pressing the chest up and down can sometimes break the ribs. Some people develop infections and other complications while being connected to a breathing machine.'

- Tell her that **the medical team feels that CPR should not be attempted if she arrests**, and explain the reasons.

'Your mother has a number of medical conditions and is quite frail, so it is very unlikely that CPR will be successful for her. We feel that it would prolong her suffering, so we should allow her to die peacefully in a dignified way if her heart stops.'

Note: Do not say that the decision to not resuscitate her was taken because of her advanced age.

- Ask for her thoughts.

'What do you feel about what I have told you?'

She says she understands what you are saying but she cannot live with the guilt that she allowed the medical team to not revive her. She finds this a bit overwhelming.

- Tell her that **it is the decision of the medical team and she does not have to feel responsible.**

'You do not have to feel responsible for this decision. The medical team has taken this decision considering her background medical problems. We feel that CPR is unlikely to be successful for her and will only prolong her suffering. We are sharing our decision with you now so that it doesn't come as a shock to you later and you know what to expect.'

She asks if this means that you won't do anything and let her die.

- Reassure her that **this does not mean that the team is giving up on her.**

'Not at all. It does not mean that we are giving up on her. She will still receive all the usual treatments for her medical conditions. We will treat her with oxygen, medicines to *remove the excess fluid from her body, antibiotics, painkillers, and medicines to reduce her suffering, if needed.*

'What this simply means is that if she reaches a point where these treatments do not work anymore and the heart stops, we will allow her to pass away naturally.'

- Tell her that the 'do not attempt cardiopulmonary resuscitation' (DNACPR) decision will be entered in her medical notes.

'We will record the decision to not resuscitate in her medical notes so that it is clear to the medical teams during future admissions.'

Note: If no DNACPR decision is made, the initial presumption should be to resuscitate.

End the discussion by summarising the main points. Reassure her once more that (1) it is the decision of the medical team to not resuscitate her, considering her multiple comorbidities and poor likelihood of success; (2) it means that we will allow her to pass away naturally instead of prolonging her suffering; (3) she does not have to feel responsible for this decision; and (4) it does not mean that we are giving up on her.

SUMMARY

This scenario tests your skills in discussing DNAR decision with the family member of a demented patient. You will be expected to:

- Explain why you wish to discuss the issue of resuscitation.
- For patients without capacity, ask the relative if the patient has ever expressed her wishes regarding extent of care.
- Check her background knowledge and ideas regarding resuscitation.
- Explain that DNACPR is the decision of the medical team and you are not seeking her consent.
- Discuss the reasons for arriving at this decision and the low likelihood of success.
- Tell her that she does not have to feel responsible for this decision.
- Reassure her that this does not mean that the team is giving up on her.

The 68-Year-Old Man with Motor Neurone Disease Who Needs Artificial Feeding

This 68-year-old man was diagnosed with motor neurone disease (MND) just over a year ago. He initially presented with weakness in his legs and frequent falls. His speech has since become increasingly slurred, and he has recently been coughing or choking while eating. The speech and language therapist (SALT) who recently assessed him felt that it was not safe for him to be fed orally.

Your task is to discuss the option of percutaneous endoscopic gastrostomy (PEG) feeding with him and his wife.

- Introduce yourself, and check the identity of the patient and his wife. Tell them that you have come to discuss about his choking. Start by asking how he is.

The wife says he is getting weaker. His speech is becoming harder to understand. Of late, he has been choking or coughing while eating. He therefore tends to eat less these days. He has lost around 3–4 kg in the last three months because of reduced food intake.

The focus of this consultation is to discuss alternative feeding options with the couple. There is no need to discuss the other aspects of his MND. Tube feeding should indeed be considered in this man, as (1) he is choking and coughing while eating, which suggests that his throat muscles are getting weaker; (2) he is at risk of aspiration pneumonia if he continues to eat by mouth; (3) he is not eating much; and (4) he has lost weight as a result. Although tube feeding will help increase his nutritional intake, it may not completely eliminate the risk of aspiration.

It is important to introduce the concept of tube feeding to the patient early in the course of the disease rather than leaving it until they become malnourished or start aspirating. Patients need time to decide, and there is often a long wait for elective procedures. Moreover, respiratory compromise during the later stages of the disease might make it challenging to administer the sedative prior to performing the procedure.

- *Ask if he has formed any ideas about his choking.* Does he realise that it is due to his MND?

He says he didn't make much of the choking. It was his wife who kept pointing out that he is eating less because of the choking. He hasn't formed any ideas about it.

DOI: 10.1201/9781003533337-46

Tell them that:

- *His dysphagia and dysarthria are due to MND.*

'*As you may have been told already, motor neurone disease damages the nerve cells that help convey messages from the brain to the muscles.*

   '*The problem now seems to be affecting the muscles around your throat, making it increasingly difficult for you to speak and swallow. This is the reason you are coughing and choking while eating. I am concerned that you have lost weight because you have not been eating much recently.*'

- *He is at risk of aspiration pneumonia.*

'*Our throat splits into two branches. One leads to the windpipe, which carries oxygen to the lungs. The other leads to the food pipe, which is located right behind the windpipe. When we swallow, the opening around the windpipe shuts to prevent food from getting into the lungs. When the throat muscles become weak, the windpipe cannot close fully. This makes it easier for food particles to get into the lungs and increase the risk of lung infection. These infections can sometimes be life-threatening.*'

- The speech and language therapist feels that *it is not safe for him to swallow.*

'*The therapist who tested your swallowing feels that it is not safe for you to eat by mouth.*'

Pause for a moment and check their understanding. Manage his emotions appropriately before proceeding ('*I can see how difficult it is for you to hear this*').

- *Introduce the concept of feeding tubes.*

'*I am afraid the swallowing problem is likely to get worse as the disease progresses, so it is important to start thinking of other ways to provide nutrition or give you the medicines. We can consider placing a feeding tube. Has anyone spoken to you about feeding tubes, or have you heard of this?*'

They say they have heard of people being fed through a tube but do not know how that works.

- *Talk to them about PEG.* Give them a brief idea of the procedure (the PEG nurse and surgeon will explain in detail later).

'*We can feed you through a special plastic tube placed directly inside your stomach. We call this gastrostomy tube, or PEG tube for short.* Gastro *refers to the stomach, and* ostomy *means opening. I'll ask our nurse to talk to you about this in detail. The procedure is performed by a surgeon.*

   '*He will make a small cut on the front part of your tummy after injecting a local anaesthetic medicine to numb the skin. You may be given a sedative medicine through the vein to make you a bit drowsy and help you relax. The feeding tube will be placed inside the stomach through this cut. A long thin tube called a scope, with a camera and light at one end, will be passed through your mouth into the stomach at the same time. The scope will help place the tube in the correct position. Once the feeding tube is secured, it'll sit on the front part of your tummy. The procedure takes less than half an hour. You should be able to go home the same day.'*

- **Discuss the benefits of PEG.**

'We can give you liquid feeds, fluids, and medicines via this tube using a syringe. A dietician will plan the composition of your feeds and ensure that you get enough nutrition.'

- **Discuss the risks of PEG.**

'There are some risks with the use of a PEG tube, which the surgeon will go through in detail before getting your consent. You may get a skin infection at the site where the tube is inserted. These infections could spread to the organs inside your belly and become serious, so it is important for anyone handling the tube to keep their hands clean. Very rarely, the tube can inadvertently create a hole in the wall of the stomach or cause excessive bleeding while it is being passed.'

- Tell them that *the risk of aspiration cannot be completely eliminated* with the use of a PEG tube.

'The PEG tube will not completely eliminate the risk of food going into the lungs, especially if you are fed too much or you are lying flat while being fed. The excess feeds or fluids can go up from the stomach into the food pipe and spill into the lungs. The nurse will teach you how to use the PEG tube. If you carefully follow her instructions, you can minimise this risk.

'All this may seem overwhelming, but please don't worry. Once you start using the tube, it'll become second nature to you.'

He asks if this means that he will never be able to taste food once the PEG is placed.

- Tell him that *he can still eat small amounts as guided by the SALT.*

'You can still eat small amounts as guided by the swallowing therapist. We call this pleasure feeding. The dietician will suggest modified feeds that are more semi-solid or liquid so that you don't choke on them. This amount may not be enough, hence the need to place the PEG tube and to ensure that your body gets enough nutrition.'

He asks if the feeding tube will remain in his stomach indefinitely.

- Tell him that *tube feeding should continue for the rest of his life.*

'Motor neurone disease is a permanent condition and one that will slowly worsen with time, so I'm afraid we must continue this method of feeding for the rest of your life. We can, of course, remove the tube anytime or not use the tube if you do not like it, although I wouldn't recommend that, because, as I said, feeding through the mouth can increase your risk of getting a lung infection, and your body won't get enough nutrition.'

He asks if there are any alternatives.

- Tell them that *nasogastric tube feeding is an alternative, but it is not ideal for long-term use*.

  'There is another type of feeding tube. It is passed through the nose and placed in the stomach. It is called a nasogastric tube. Having the tube in the nose is not very comfortable, so we do not use this tube for more than a few weeks. It is not ideal for long-term use. There is a risk of the food getting into the lungs with the use of this method of feeding too.'

End the discussion by summarising the main points. Tell them that once they have made up their mind, you will refer him to a PEG nurse, who will explain the procedure and the practical aspects in further detail. Ask them to get in touch with you if they have any queries in the meantime. Tell them that you will give them written information or details of some useful websites.

Most patients do not like the idea of tube feeding and may resist it when they are first introduced to the idea. If he refuses, tell him that you will be happy to arrange another appointment to discuss this or you would ask the nurse to speak to them about this. (*'I understand. We can discuss this again in a few days, or I can ask the nurse to talk to you. I would recommend doing this fairly soon, as you are already choking while eating, and we don't want you to end up getting a lung infection.'*)

SUMMARY

This scenario tests your skills in discussing alternative feeding options for a patient with an incurable neurological illness. You will be expected to:

- Explain to him that his swallowing is unsafe due to the progression of his motor neurone disease.
- Explain that he is at risk of aspiration pneumonia if he continues to eat by mouth.
- Introduce the concept of PEG feeding.

Briefly discuss how the procedure is performed and its benefits, risks, and alternatives.

- Tell him that the risk of aspiration cannot be completely eliminated with PEG feeding.
- Reassure him that he can still eat a small amount of food by mouth for pleasure, as guided by the swallowing therapist.
- Tell him that tube feeding will be continued for the rest of his life unless he changes his mind later.

The 70-Year-Old Man with Acute Exacerbation of COPD

This 70-year-old man, with a background history of chronic obstructive pulmonary disease (COPD), hypertension, hyperlipidaemia, and benign prostate enlargement, was admitted last night with a three-day history of worsening of his breathlessness and change in the colour of the sputum to yellow.

His chest X-ray revealed changes of COPD and some haziness in the right lower zone. Blood test results showed elevated white blood cell count and neutrophilia. His blood glucose, liver, and renal function were normal. He was diagnosed with acute infective exacerbation of COPD and commenced on nebulised bronchodilators, corticosteroids, intravenous amoxicillin–clavulanic acid, and oxygen via Venturi mask.

He initially seemed to respond to the treatments. However, he has become increasingly drowsy since this morning. His vital signs recorded a little earlier showed normal temperature, oxygen saturation 90% on 50% oxygen by Venturi mask, pulse rate 98/minute, respiratory rate 24/minute, and blood pressure 136/88 mmHg. His arterial blood gases revealed respiratory acidosis, with pO_2 11.2 kPa (normal 11–14 kPa), pCO_2 8.4 kPa (normal 4.5–6.5 kPa), and pH 7.21 (normal 7.35–7.45).

Your consultant feels that invasive ventilation should be considered because of the respiratory acidosis and increasing drowsiness. He has asked you to talk to his daughter, who has just arrived.

- Introduce yourself, and confirm the identity and relationship of the daughter. Tell her that you have come to update her about her father.

She says she just saw her father. He was drowsy and unable to recognise her. Although he was breathless at the time of admission, he was not drowsy. He was still managing to talk to her in short sentences last night. She wants to know why he has become drowsy. She says she is worried.

DOI: 10.1201/9781003533337-47

- Say something reassuring, and *find out what she has been told already*.

  'I can see that you are worried. We are doing our best to help him. Before I explain why he has become drowsy and what we plan to do next, may I find out what you have been told about your father's lung condition and the reason for his current illness?'

She says her father has had this lung problem for many years. She is not sure what exactly it is called, but he gets a lung infection from time to time, especially during the winter months. He gets more breathless at those times and starts coughing up mucky phlegm that would look green or yellow. He always responds to a course of an antibiotic, the name of which she cannot recall.

He had a similar flare-up two to three days ago and started taking the antibiotic given by the GP, but it wasn't helpful this time. His breathing continued to worsen, so she decided to bring him to the hospital last night. He was started on oxygen and given some medicine through the mask and another one through the vein. She says he has never been drowsy like this before.

Tell her that:

- *Her father's illness is due to an exacerbation of his chronic lung condition.*

  'We breathe in oxygen and breathe out carbon dioxide. The oxygen that we breathe in passes through the windpipe and then through the airways in both the lungs. The problem with your father's lungs is that the airways are narrow. The muscles around the airways are tight. The lining of the airways is inflamed and swollen. The air is not able to freely move in and out because of the narrowing. The problem has been made worse by the infection in his lungs.'

Note: She mainly wants to know why her father is drowsy and what you plan to do next. There is no need to specifically state that his underlying diagnosis is COPD or that the problem was caused by his smoking habit.

Even if you decide to state the diagnosis, say that in the end as: '*We call this chronic obstructive pulmonary disease. Chronic means long-standing.* Obstructive *because there is an obstruction to the free flow of air through the lungs.* Pulmonary *refers to the lungs.'* Do not start with this: '*Your father's lung condition is called chronic obstructive pulmonary disease. I know it's a bit of a mouthful.'*

- *You are treating him with bronchodilators, corticosteroid, and antibiotics.*

  'Apart from oxygen, we are giving him medicines through the mask to open the breathing tubes. We are giving him a steroid medicine to reduce the swelling in the lining of the airways, and an antibiotic through the vein to treat the infection.'

- *He is drowsy most likely because of carbon dioxide retention.*

  'I'm afraid he is not responding well to these treatments. The narrowing of the airways is making it difficult for him to breathe out the carbon dioxide. He is getting drowsy

because of the carbon dioxide that is accumulating in the blood. Giving him oxygen alone is therefore not helping. We must also do something to remove the carbon dioxide.'

Pause for a moment and check her understanding (*'Do you understand what I have told you so far? Is there anything you want me to repeat?'*) Invite any questions.

She says she understands. She asks what you can do to remove the carbon dioxide.

- Tell her that **the consultant has suggested mechanical ventilation.**

  'My consultant has suggested that we connect him to a breathing machine. The breathing machine will not only provide oxygen but also remove the excess carbon dioxide that is accumulating in his blood. It involves passing a tube down his throat before connecting him to the machine. We'll have to shift him to the intensive care unit if we decide to proceed with this.'

Before explaining further, you should check:

- **If he has ever expressed his wishes about how he should be managed if he became ill** or made an advance decision to refuse treatment (ADRT).

  'Has he ever told you that he wouldn't want to be connected to a breathing machine or have anything else aggressive done if he became severely ill?'

- **His comorbidities.**

Confirm that he is not known to have any medical problems apart from hypertension, hyperlipidaemia, and benign prostate enlargement.

- **His overall quality of life.**

How was his day-to-day life? Was he ambulant? Was he able to manage his daily chores without assistance? How was his mental state?

- **If he has ever been in an intensive care unit** (ICU).

She says he has never discussed his views, either verbally or in writing, on how he should be treated if he became severely ill. He did not have any other medical problems apart from the ones you mentioned.

He used to be a gardener, until he stopped working more than ten years ago. He lives with her mum, and they both manage the daily chores between them. He is still ambulant, although he walks a bit slowly at his own pace. Apart from the times when his lung condition flares up, he is not too bad. There is no problem with his mental functions. He has never been in the ICU.

There is no ADRT, and he has never expressed his wishes verbally about how he should be treated if he became ill. We should therefore treat him in his best interests. Given that his pre-morbid quality of life and function were reasonable, we should proceed with mechanical ventilation.

- Tell her that *you would recommend mechanical ventilation,* as his pre-morbid quality of life was good and he never expressed a wish to refuse such treatments.

'I asked you those questions because not everyone will benefit from a breathing machine. Some people are unlikely to recover even if they are connected to the machine, and it may simply prolong their suffering. As your father did not have too many medical problems, I feel that we should go ahead with our plan and connect him to the breathing machine. It'll give him the best chance for recovery. I am hoping that he won't need the breathing machine for more than a few days.'

She says she understands and concurs with your plan to connect him to the ventilator. She asks how ill he is and if he is likely to die.

- Tell her that *he is critically ill and there is a chance that he could die.*

'Your father is quite unwell at present. I think we should be prepared for the worst, but we are trying to do all that we can to make sure he recovers.'

Note: This is one of the most difficult questions to answer! There are many different ways to respond, but this sentence has conveyed to her that there is a chance that he might die, and it is quickly followed by the second part, which conveys some hope and gives her the reassurance that we are doing our best. She says her brother lives in Australia, and wonders if she should ask him to come over.

- Tell her that *it is difficult to predict his outcome,* but it may be a good idea to ask him to come over.

'It is a bit difficult to predict how he will respond to the treatments. You can tell your brother that your father is quite unwell and things could go either way. He should not regret later that he did not get the chance to see your father, in case he does not respond well to the treatments, so it may be a good idea for him to come over if he is able to. You'll need his support as well during this very difficult time.'

End the conversation by asking about her mother. Summarise the main points, and tell her what will happen next. (*'We will shorty take him down to the ICU. The doctor in the ICU will explain further about the breathing machine.'*) Tell her that she can ask to speak to you if she has any further questions before he is taken down to the ICU.

SUMMARY

This scenario tests your skills in discussing the management plan with the daughter of a seriously ill patient. You will be expected to:

- Find out what the daughter has already been told about her father's illness.

- Explain that his illness is due to exacerbation of his underlying chronic lung condition, and outline the treatments given so far.
- Tell her that he is drowsy because of rising pCO_2.
- Discuss the option of mechanical ventilation.
- Ask relevant questions to check his pre-morbid quality of life and comorbidities.
- Ask if he has ever expressed his wishes, either verbally or in writing, about how he should be managed if he became severely ill.

Note: You will receive an unsatisfactory mark if you do not check his pre-morbid quality of life or ask if he has ever expressed his wishes.

- Tell her that there is a chance that he could die but you are doing your best to get him well.

The 81-Year-Old Man Who Is Terminally Ill

This 81-year-old man, with a background history of metastatic prostate cancer (for which he declined treatment), diabetes mellitus, hypertension, hyperlipidaemia, chronic kidney disease stage 3, and ischaemic heart disease, was admitted ten days ago with right lower lobe pneumonia.

Despite receiving piperacillin–tazobactam, his oxygen requirement has remained high at 15 L/minute by non-rebreather mask (NRM), and his most recent chest X-ray, done yesterday, showed worsening consolidation. His kidney function, which acutely declined during this admission, has not improved much either. He has become increasingly drowsy and just been commenced on fentanyl and hyoscine to reduce his respiratory distress and secretions. The medical team placed a 'do not attempt resuscitation' order at the time of admission, and his family is aware of this. There was no 'advance care plan' discussion in the past, so his wishes are not known.

The consultant feels that it is time to stop the antibiotics and intravenous fluids, as he is terminally ill, with no prospect of recovery. She feels that he should be referred to the palliative team and kept comfortable until he dies naturally. Your task is to discuss this with the son and daughter. You can assume that they know you well, as you have been part of the medical team taking care of their father for the last ten days.

- Start by greeting the son and daughter. Tell them that you have come to update them on their father's progress. Ask them to recap what they have been told so far.

The son says he understands that his father is seriously ill with a lung infection and his kidneys are not working well. He and his sister are grateful to the team for all the care they are providing. Although they have not seen any improvement in his health condition since bringing him to the hospital ten days ago, they are hoping that he will respond to the treatments and show some progress.

Tell them that:

- *He has not responded well to the treatments.*

  'I'm afraid I don't have very good news for you. The chest X-ray that was done yesterday shows that his lung infection is worsening. He is still requiring a very high amount

DOI: 10.1201/9781003533337-48

of oxygen, and we haven't been able to reduce it at all. His kidneys have not improved either.

'As you know, we have been treating him with a strong antibiotic for the last ten days. He has unfortunately not responded to our treatments, and his progress overall has been disappointing. We have done everything possible to help him, but his advanced age and the multiple medical problems are making it harder for him to fight the infection.'

- **You would like to discuss the next steps.**

'As he has not responded to the treatments and his condition is getting worse, we must now decide what to do next.'

- The medical team feels that *it is best to shift to comfort care.*

'I am afraid he is very close to the end of his life. [Pause for a moment.] We feel that it is not in his best interests to continue the antibiotic. Continuing the treatments in an attempt to cure the lung infection is not going to work. It will only prolong his suffering and distress. Rather than prolonging life, these treatments may simply be delaying his death. We therefore wonder if we should shift our focus from trying to cure the pneumonia to making sure he is comfortable and does not suffer.'

The son says he is very sad to hear that his father hasn't responded to the treatments. He says they are not bold enough to make the decision to stop the antibiotic. They wouldn't be able to live with that guilt for the rest of their lives.

Tell them that:

- **It is the decision of the medical team to withdraw treatment.**

'I am sorry if I did not make that clear. You do not have to feel pressured into making that decision. The medical team has taken this decision based on his background medical problems, severity of the lung infection, and lack of response to the antibiotic. We are only seeking your concurrence.'

- **You are not withdrawing care.**

'Stopping the treatments for his lung infection does not mean that we are going to stop caring for him.'

- **The team will make sure he does not suffer.**

'We will continue to provide the necessary treatments to ensure that he does not suffer. We have just started him on medications to make his breathing easier and reduce the secretions in his throat. We will also ask the palliative team to see him. The palliative doctors and nurses are experts in providing care towards the end of life.'

- *You would recommend stopping the intravenous fluids as well.*

'We would also recommend stopping the drip and not giving any more fluids. It'll reduce the secretions in his throat and ensure that he does not get overloaded with fluids. It'll help to further improve his comfort.'

The son says he is concerned that you are withdrawing fluids, especially as he is already not being fed. Would he not die from starvation and dehydration? he asks.

- *Explain why you are not feeding him.*

'He will die because of the lung infection, not from starvation or dehydration. Feeding him at this stage is dangerous. As he is drowsy, the food could go down the wrong path into the lungs and make matters worse. Not receiving feeds or fluids will not hasten his death or add to his distress. If we stop the fluids, his mouth and lips could become dry, but we'll make sure we regularly moisten them.'

Clinically assisted nutrition refers to nutrition provided via a nasogastric tube, percutaneous endoscopic gastrostomy, or the parenteral route, while *clinically assisted hydration* refers to the administration of fluids, either intravenously or subcutaneously.

Although the issue of withdrawing nutrition and hydration in a dying patient is contentious and subject to debate, it is not considered euthanasia or unethical. Feeding and hydration towards the end of life are associated with the risk of aspiration, nausea, vomiting, diarrhoea, fluid overload, and increased throat secretions. It is, however, prudent to get the concurrence of the family members and check their cultural or religious beliefs before deciding to withdraw nutrition and hydration.

After some reluctance, the son concurs with the decision of the medical team to stop the antibiotics and fluids. He asks if he can be discharged so that he can die at home.

- Check the reasons for this request. *Ask if their dad has ever expressed a wish to die at home* and what the home circumstances are like. What kind of accommodation is it? Who can take care of him at home?

His dad has never expressed such a wish, but he knows that that is what he would have preferred. When his mother was terminally ill ten years ago, his dad was keen for her to be brought home just before she died. She, however, died in the hospital, and that upset him a lot. He says he will take his dad to his house, which is only 2 miles away. He can place a bed in the living room downstairs. He and his two sisters will take turns taking care of him.

- *Briefly explain the process of terminal discharge.*

'We sometimes do, indeed, discharge terminally ill patients so that they can peacefully die at home in their familiar surroundings, but this may not suit everyone. Sadly, some patients die in the ambulance on their way home. We can arrange for a hospice or a *district nurse to check on him daily, but a majority of the care should still be provided by the family members. This may involve giving him injections, sponging him, changing his diapers, and performing oral hygiene. We will train you to perform all these tasks and also manage his symptoms, like agitation, pain, breathing difficulty, and throat secretions. It is not possible to predict how long he will live, so you and your family members must be prepared to perform these tasks, even if it extends to several days.'*

- Tell them that he is on high-flow oxygen, which can be challenging to continue at home.

'He is still receiving 15 litres of oxygen per minute via a special mask, which is not easy to continue at home. It is possible to get an oxygen concentrator at home, but this may not be able to provide 15 litres per minute. However, over the next several hours, we can try to gradually reduce the oxygen and see how he gets on with that. Reducing the oxygen will not hasten his death or cause any discomfort. I will ask the palliative doctor to discuss this further with you.'

- Encourage the family to spend as much time as possible with the patient.

'We realise that this is a very difficult time for your whole family. Try to spend as much time as possible with your father. Please think about the challenges that I mentioned in taking him home.'

End the conversation by summarising the main points and what you have agreed on. Tell them that (1) the team will stop the antibiotic and withdraw the fluids as he has responded poorly to the treatments, (2) the team will continue to care for him and make sure he receives appropriate interventions to reduce his distress, and (3) you will revisit the issue of terminal discharge once they have made up their mind.

SUMMARY

This scenario tests your skills in discussing the withdrawal of treatment for a terminally ill patient. You will be expected to tell the son and daughter that:

- The clinical condition of their father is worsening, and he is likely to die soon.
- The focus should shift from trying to cure the pneumonia to ensuring that he is kept comfortable and does not suffer.
- The team would like to stop the antibiotics, withdraw fluids, and continue with palliative measures alone.
- Withdrawal of treatment does not equate to withdrawal of care.
- There are some challenges in terminally discharging him.

You should appropriately respond to the emotions of the son and daughter throughout the consultation.

The 45-Year-Old Man with Severe Brain Haemorrhage

This 45-year-old man was brought to the hospital a couple of hours ago after he collapsed at work during a meeting. He clutched his head before he slumped on the table. He was previously in good health, with no known medical problems.

He was comatose upon arrival at the emergency department. Computed tomography scan of his brain showed extensive subarachnoid haemorrhage extending into the ventricles. The consultant neurosurgeon, who came to see him straightaway, ruled out an operative intervention because of the extent of bleeding.

He has been shifted to the intensive care unit (ICU) and connected to a mechanical ventilator. The clinical impression of the ICU team is that he is most likely brain-dead, but they have asked two senior clinicians to formally confirm this. They have also requested the appropriate blood tests to rule out reversible causes of brainstem injury. Your task is to speak to the wife, who has just arrived.

As soon as you enter the room, a woman in her late 30s hurriedly asks you how her husband is. She is extremely anxious and distressed.

- First, introduce yourself and make sure you are talking to the correct person (in real life, make sure you take a nurse with you).

Even before you start talking further, she says she received a phone call from her husband's colleague. She only told her that he was taken to the hospital in an ambulance after collapsing at work. She did not tell her anything else. She asks if her husband is OK and where he is. Gently break the news after a warning shot. Speak slowly and clearly in short sentences.

- Tell her that *her husband has suffered a massive brain haemorrhage.*

'*I am sorry, but I have some bad news to share. Your husband [mention his first name] has suffered a massive brain haemorrhage.*'

DOI: 10.1201/9781003533337-49

Do not continue talking after this. Give her some time. Respond appropriately to her emotions. Then tell her (with appropriate pauses along the way) that:

- *He has been connected to a ventilator and taken to the intensive care unit.*

  'His brain scan showed extensive bleeding in and around the brain. He was unconscious when he was brought to the hospital. He was not able to breathe on his own, so we have connected him to a breathing machine. He is now in the intensive care unit.'

- *The neurosurgeon has ruled out operative intervention.*

  'The brain surgeon came to see him straightaway. He feels that an operation to remove the blood will not be feasible, as the bleeding is quite extensive.'

- *He has suffered severe brain damage because of the haemorrhage.*

  'We feel that his brain is severely damaged because of the bleeding. I am so sorry.'

It is not easy for a young woman to accept the shocking news that her husband, who was previously in good health, has suffered a massive brain haemorrhage, causing severe brain damage. It is difficult for anyone in a highly emotional state to comprehend this properly, so you might have to repeat yourself if she asks questions like 'Why is he on a breathing machine?' 'Why can't you remove the blood from the brain?' or 'Where is he now?' When you answer these questions, do not start the sentence with 'As I just told you'.

There are two mistakes to avoid at this stage:

1. Do not say that he is brain-dead (that is only the impression of the clinical team).

You cannot say that he is brain-dead yet, as there are strict criteria for its diagnosis. It must be separately confirmed and certified by two clinicians who are not part of the treating team. Moreover, reversible causes should be ruled out first (e.g. toxins, metabolic derangements, hypothermia). Not all patients with brain damage are brain-dead.

2. Do not discuss organ donation.

Even after he is certified as brain-dead, it is insensitive to discuss organ donation before she has come to terms with the news.

In real life, the next part of the conversation usually takes place at a later stage, but in an exam setting, the actor will be trained to quickly recover from the shocking news and ask you some questions.

She says this is overwhelming for her. She asks if there is even a slim chance that he will recover.

Tell her that:

- *Two clinicians will do some tests to check his brainstem function.*

  '*I can see how difficult it is for you to take all this in. Two senior doctors will now come and separately do some tests on him. These tests will tell us if there is damage to the brainstem, which is the part of the brain that helps us breathe. We've also asked for a number of blood tests to rule out other conditions that can affect the brainstem.*'

- *If the tests conclude that he is brain-dead, there is no chance of recovery at all.*

  '*If the tests show that his brainstem is permanently damaged and the blood tests rule out other causes, there is no chance for recovery at all. He won't be able to breathe without the support of the breathing machine. Once the breathing machine is turned off, the heart will stop beating shortly afterwards. We call this brain death. If he is pronounced brain-dead, it means he has died.*'

She gets extremely upset when you tell her that there is a chance that he has possibly died. She asks what those tests entail and how soon they can be done.

- *Briefly tell her about the process of diagnosing brain death.*

  '*They will carefully go through a number of steps to find out if he is brain-dead. They will turn off the breathing machine for a short period to see if he is making any attempt to breathe on his own. They'll also do a few other tests, like touching the front part of his eye with cotton wool to see if he blinks, shining a torch into both eyes to see if they react to light, tickling the back of the throat to see if he coughs, and so forth.*
  '*It may take some time to complete all the necessary tests, because we must be absolutely certain that he is brain-dead. If the tests do not give a clear answer, they will be repeated after some time. If the tests are not conclusive, the intensive care doctors may ask for a special brain scan and a tracing of the brain. If he is brain-dead, the scan will show no blood flow to the brain and the tracing will show no electrical activity in the brain.*'

She says he was health-conscious and went for his annual health checks without fail. He had no medical problems at all. She wonders how someone like him could have developed this problem.

- Tell her that *the most likely cause is a ruptured cerebral aneurysm*.

  '*Some people develop a weakness in the blood vessel wall which causes it to bulge. We call this an aneurysm. This kind of bleeding occurs when the bulged part of the blood vessel in the brain bursts. Brain aneurysms can develop in anyone. There is nothing that he could have done to prevent this.*'

She says he was very well until that morning. She asks if he would have had any symptoms prior to that morning that they might have possibly missed.

- After checking if he ever complained of headaches in the past, tell her that *most patients with subarachnoid haemorrhage do not experience any warning symptoms* (e.g. sentinel headache).

'*A small number of people with brain aneurysms may develop a headache during the days to weeks preceding a major bleed. This is due to small leaks from the blood vessels in the brain. In most people with this kind of bleeding, however, it happens suddenly, without any warning.*'

If she has no further questions:

- *Ask about her family.*

She says they have two children, aged 10 and 12. She feels distraught and says she is not sure how she is going to deliver this news to them.

- After saying some comforting words, tell her that someone will take her to the ICU so that she can see her husband. The ICU team will continue to update her regularly.

A person is said to have died when there is irreversible loss of cardiopulmonary function *or* irreversible loss of all brain functions. Someone who is brain-dead is clinically and legally dead once certified by two independent senior clinicians. The time when the second clinican certifies brain death will be recorded as the time of death. Relatives may become confused if this is not conveyed clearly, especially when organ donation is discussed. They should not think that organs are taken out while the person is alive and the ventilator is turned off afterwards. They should clearly be told that death will be declared *before* the organs are retrieved (declaration of death, followed by retrieval of organs, followed by the turning off of the ventilator).

Organ donation should be discussed only after he is pronounced brain-dead, *never before that*. Countries have different laws, so the way organ donation is discussed will depend on whether the country where you live has an opt-in or opt-out system. In the opt-in system, adults with mental capacity can voluntarily register as an organ donor (they will carry a donor card). The problem is that if the person did not opt in during life, family members may not know what they would have preferred. They are likely to take the safest course of action, which is to refuse organ donation. In the opt-out system, doctors will remove the organs from every brain-dead person unless they opted out during life.

Thus, consent is explicit in the opt-in system and presumed in the opt-out system. It is called 'hard' opt-in or opt-out if relatives cannot object to the removal of organs, and 'soft' opt-in or opt-out if the doctor decides not to remove the organs if faced with opposition from relatives. It can be extremely challenging even for the most seasoned clinician if the family opposes organ donation in a country with a hard opt-out system *or* they go against the wishes of the deceased person who registered to be an organ donor in a country with an opt-in system.

Once all reversible causes have been excluded and two senior clinicians have confirmed brain death, the wife should be told: '*The senior doctors have completed the tests. I am sorry to say that they have confirmed that the brainstem is permanently damaged. There is no chance for recovery. This means your husband has died.*'

The topic of organ donation should then be gently broached at the right moment. This is usually done by the ICU team and transplant coordinators. Regardless of whether there is an opt-in or opt-out system in place, it is best to start with '*What do you think about organ donation? Did your husband have any views about that?*' before explaining, '*Although the brain is damaged, the other organs are still working with the help of artificial support. His heart, liver, two kidneys, and corneas, which are the clear part on the front of the eyes, can be donated to suitable recipients before we turn off the breathing machine.*'

It should be clarified that the body will be treated with utmost respect, and care will be taken to not disfigure the person during the process of organ retrieval. The incisions made will be similar to those done on living people. The family members should be thanked profusely for the noble deed, which will enable four people to live longer and two people to get their eyesight back.

SUMMARY

This scenario tests your skills in breaking the bad news of massive cerebral haemorrhage to a young wife and discussing the issues around brain death. You will be expected to:

- Gently break the bad news that the husband has suffered a massive brain haemorrhage.
- Provide emotional management.
- Tell her that the likely cause of the brain haemorrhage is a ruptured cerebral aneurysm.
- Tell her that two clinicians will separately assess him to check if he is brain-dead, and blood tests will be done to rule out reversible causes.
- Briefly explain how brain death will be confirmed.
- Make it very clear that once he is pronounced brain-dead, he will be considered dead and no recovery is possible.

The 59-Year-Old Man Who Has Just Died from Myocardial Infarction

This 59-year-old man was brought by his wife to the emergency department around three o'clock this morning, which was just over an hour ago. His wife said he woke up complaining of central chest pain, breathlessness, and nausea.

He only spoke a couple of short sentences when he was transferred from the trolley to the bed ('*I am a diabetic*', '*I want to throw up*'). He was profusely sweating at that time. His oxygen saturation was 89% on room air, pulse rate 108/minute and regular, respiratory rate 28/minute, and blood pressure 88/60 mmHg. Fine crackles were heard throughout his lung fields. His 12-lead electro-cardiogram showed extensive anterolateral ST segment elevation.

He was commenced on oxygen, given furosemide, and loaded with aspirin. The on-call cardiologist was informed, and the cardiac catheterisation lab was activated straightaway. However, within minutes of arrival, he developed generalised tonic–clonic seizures that lasted about 30 seconds, most likely due to cerebral hypoperfusion. As soon as the seizures aborted, he became pulseless and stopped breathing. The monitor showed ventricular fibrillation. The cardiac arrest team, which included doctors from the intensive care unit, arrived promptly. He was defibrillated thrice, but the rhythm soon turned into asystole. He was pronounced dead after a further 45 minutes of cardiopulmonary resuscitation (CPR).

His wife is in the visitor's room. When she was last updated, soon after arrival, she was told that her husband has suffered a heart attack and arrangements were being made to perform a procedure. She is not aware that he suffered a cardiac arrest. Your task is to break the news of her husband's death to her. You are the medical registrar.

Introduce yourself, and confirm her identity. You must be absolutely certain that you are talking to the correct person when breaking a news like this.

- *Gently break the news to her after a warning shot and a momentary pause.*

'*I am sorry, but I have very bad news. [After a momentary pause.] Your husband has died.*'

DOI: 10.1201/9781003533337-50

Note: Clearly say 'died'. Do not use euphemisms or ambiguous terms like 'passed away', 'passed on', 'gone', 'no more', 'expired', 'no longer with us', 'we failed to save him', or 'we have lost him'.

Do not continue talking after this or just say: '*We tried our best but could not revive him. I am so sorry.*' Give her time. Play it by ear and see how she responds.

Breaking the death news of a family member is among the most stressful things that doctors (and military and police officers) do. It is particularly difficult when the death is sudden or unexpected. It is very hard to see someone going through that grief, and our efforts should be directed towards supporting them.

You must know the sequence of events before death very well before walking into the room. It is important to speak slowly and clearly, provide the information in small chunks, avoid medical jargon, repeat important points, make sure she understood what you said, allow moments of silence, and not interrupt her when she talks.

In real life, the discussion that follows will usually happen several minutes after breaking the bad news, but in the exam setting, the actor will be asked to recover quickly and ask you some questions.

She starts talking after a minute or so. She tells you that he was absolutely fine the previous evening and went to bed at the usual time, around 10:30 p.m. He woke her up at 2:30 a.m., complaining that he had chest pain and trouble breathing. He was profusely sweating at that time. She was worried that the ambulance may not arrive on time, so she drove him to the hospital herself. She says she is unable to accept this news, as he was generally fit and well. He had no medical problems apart from diabetes.

She asks you to narrate what happened after you took him inside and how he died. She laments that she wished she were by his side when he breathed his last.

Tell her (with appropriate pauses along the way) that:

- *He died from myocardial infarction.*

  '*He had a massive heart attack. A heart attack occurs when a blood clot blocks a blood vessel that supplies the heart muscle. Blood stops flowing through the blocked blood vessel and damages the heart muscle. His heart attack was caused by blockage of a large blood vessel, so the damage was too extensive, and it made his heart very weak.*'

- *He was critically ill and arrested within a few minutes.*

  '*He was quite unwell when he arrived. His blood pressure was very low, and there was fluid in his lungs. We connected him to oxygen. We gave him medicines to improve the blood flow to the heart muscle and remove the fluid from his lungs. We informed the heart specialist straightaway so that he could perform a procedure to open the blocked blood vessel.*

  '*Unfortunately, when we were preparing him to have this procedure, he developed fits. We believe that the fits occurred because there was not enough blood flowing to the brain. The fits lasted about 30 seconds. Right after that, his heart stopped suddenly. We initiated resuscitation at once. We pressed his chest up and down to keep the blood moving. We gave shocks to his chest and injected medicines to try to restart the heart. We used a bag to expand his lungs and provide oxygen. We tried our best for more than 45 minutes but could not revive him.'*

- **You could not get her to be by his side when he died, as his heart stopped suddenly.**

'I am sorry that you could not be present by his side when he died, but his heart stopped suddenly right after he had the fits. We could not call you inside or come out and talk to you, as we were all focused on trying to bring him back to life.'

Why was there fluid in the lungs? she asks.

- Tell her that *acute pulmonary oedema is a complication of acute myocardial infarction.*

'When the heart muscle becomes too weak, it increases the pressure in the lungs and forces the fluid into the airways. We gave him plenty of oxygen and a medicine to remove the fluid from the lungs.'

She asks if he would have suffered.

- Tell her that *he was unconscious from the time he had the seizures.*

'We acted very quickly as soon as he arrived to make him feel better. He was unconscious from the time he had the fits, so he wouldn't have felt any pain or distress after the first few minutes of arriving here.'

She says she felt confident that he was in safe hands from the minute they arrived in the hospital but now feels let down. She asks if it would have made a difference if the cardiologist had been physically present in the hospital at the time when her husband arrived.

- Tell her *that he was managed appropriately and the team tried their best.* Reassure her that he received the best possible care. This is important for her to get closure.

'We tried our best to save him, but the damage to his heart was too great. I want to reassure you that we did everything that had to be done. All of us in the team have the necessary skills and experience to manage people who are critically ill.
  'We informed the heart specialist straightaway, and he was on his way to the hospital to perform the procedure. Even if he had been here at the time when your husband arrived, he wouldn't have been able to perform the procedure, as his heart stopped within a few minutes of arriving here.'

She asks if she should have called the ambulance instead of driving him to the hospital herself.

- Reassure her that *it would not have changed the final outcome.*

'I think you did whatever you thought was correct at that time. Please don't blame yourself. At this time of the night, you probably took the same amount of time that the ambulance would have taken to get him here. His heart did not stop on the way to the hospital, so the ambulance personnel wouldn't have done anything different. They would

have connected him to oxygen and given him the blood-thinning tablet earlier, but that wouldn't have changed the final outcome.'

- If she has no further questions, ***ask about her family***.

She says she has two daughters. They live in a neighbouring town. She told them over the phone soon after arriving in the hospital that she has brought their father to the hospital. They are both on their way to the hospital.

End the conversation by conveying your condolences. Tell her that the nurse will shortly take her to see her husband. Ask her to not hesitate to ask you or anyone in the team if she needs any help.

SUMMARY

Although acute myocardial infarction is not unexpected in a 59-year-old diabetic man, the sudden death of a close family member is extremely difficult for anyone to accept. You will be expected to:

- Gently break the bad news after a warning shot.
- Respond to her emotions appropriately.
- Clearly narrate the sequence of events in layman's terms but do not give too much information all at once.
- Reassure her that the team did their best and the physical presence of the cardiologist would not have made a difference.
- Tell her that she should not blame herself for not calling the ambulance, as it would not have changed the final outcome.

The 53-Year-Old Woman Whose Death Is Unexplained

This 53-year-old woman was brought to the emergency department (ED) by her husband about three hours ago as she complained of chest and abdominal discomfort at home. She only spoke through sign language, as she was deaf from birth. Her medical history was otherwise unremarkable, and she did not take any regular medication.

She could not give any history to the ED doctor but kept making circular motions with her hand pointing to her chest and abdomen. She was sweating profusely and appeared to be in some kind of distress. Her temperature was 36.2°C, oxygen saturation 96% on room air, pulse rate 102/minute, respiratory rate 28/minute, and blood pressure 150/98 mmHg. There was no difference in blood pressure between the two arms. Her heart sounds were normal, and lungs were clear. Abdomen was soft and non-tender. Her 12-lead electrocardiogram and capillary blood glucose were normal. The ED doctor asked for a chest X-ray and planned to do a bedside ultrasound scan of her abdomen. His admission diagnosis was 'panic attack'.

A few minutes after the initial assessment and before any of the imaging investigations could be carried out, she was suddenly found unresponsive by the nurse. Cardiopulmonary resuscitation (CPR) was initiated straightaway as she was pulseless and not breathing. The cardiac monitor showed asystole. She was pronounced dead after 50 minutes of CPR. Blood samples that were drawn before she arrested showed that her blood counts, liver function tests, serum creatinine, urea and electrolytes, amylase, D-dimer, and troponin were all normal.

The husband has already been told that she has died. Your task is to now inform him that you will be referring to the coroner, as the cause of her death is unexplained. You are the medical registrar on call.

Introduce yourself, and confirm his relationship to the deceased. Make sure you are talking to the correct person.

- Start by expressing your condolences on the passing away of his wife. Briefly ask what happened at home before he brought her to hospital and *what he has been told about her death.*

DOI: 10.1201/9781003533337-51

He says his wife was in good health, with no major medical issues. She seldom saw a doctor during the 30 years that he had been married to her. She was not taking any regular medication. She never smoked or drank alcohol.

They were sitting on the sofa at home, watching television, when she suddenly expressed to him in sign language that she was not feeling comfortable. He decided to bring her to the hospital as she kept pointing to her chest and tummy. He says he is deeply shocked and did not expect her to die. The doctor who conveyed the news of her death told him that the team was not sure why she died, as everything happened very quickly.

Tell him that:

- *The cause of her death is unexplained.*

  'Yes, we are not sure what caused her death. Heart attack, a large blood clot in the lung, a tear on the inner lining of the big blood vessel that leaves the heart, and losing a lot of blood internally are some of the possible causes for someone to develop chest or tummy pain and die so suddenly. However, we did not find any evidence of those conditions when we examined her.

  'Her heartbeat and breathing were faster. Her blood pressure was a little high, and she was sweating profusely. There was otherwise nothing else abnormal to find. The tracing of her heart and the blood test results were all normal. We, too, did not expect her heart to stop so suddenly. I am sorry that despite our best efforts, we could not revive her.'

- [After a brief pause] **You will not be able to complete the medical certificate of the cause of death** (MCCD), as the cause of her death is not known.

  'When someone dies, we normally complete a certificate that states the cause of death. You need this certificate to register her death and get the death certificate. I'm afraid we won't be able to complete that certificate for her, as we do not know what caused her death.'

- *You will have to refer to the coroner.*

  'We must therefore refer her to a coroner. We refer all unexplained deaths to the coroner. A coroner is a judicial officer who works with the police and a medical expert called a pathologist. They'll try to establish the cause of death when doctors are unable to do so.'

The husband gets upset when you mention the word 'police'. 'Why do you have to refer to the police?' he asks.

- Tell him that the coroner works with the police as *some unexplained deaths are not due to natural causes.*

  'They work as a team. The police officer is part of their team, as some of the deaths that are reported to the coroner are not due to natural causes. He might ask to speak to you and some of us in the medical team to find out what happened. For most cases, the coroner and the pathologist will go through the medical notes and conclude that the death is *due to a natural cause. If the coroner is unable to determine the cause of death, he might ask for a post-mortem to be performed.'*

The MCCD can be completed only if (1) the identity of the person is known, (2) the cause of death can be established, *and* (3) the death is due to a natural cause (all three). A coroner's referral should be made if (1) the identity of the person is unknown, (2) the deceased was not attended by a medical practitioner during the last two weeks prior to death, *or* (3) the death is unexplained, unnatural (e.g. suicide, related to accident or trauma), suspicious, iatrogenic (e.g. related to a drug, procedure, surgery, or anaesthetic), or custodial (e.g. death of a person in prison or police custody). The family can also approach the coroner if they suspect that the death was due to lapse in medical care.

The coroner must establish who died and when, where, and how the death occurred. The coroner will decide if (1) the cause of death is natural, (2) a post-mortem examination is required, or (3) an inquest should be opened. The coroner will open an inquest if the cause of death is not clear even after the post-mortem examination, the death is unnatural or due to lapse of care, or the person died while in custody. An inquest is an inquiry, which may be followed by a court hearing to establish the facts about the circumstances of the death.

The husband asks if it is possible to find out the cause of her death without doing a post-mortem.

- *Ask if there is a religious reason for his request* (an important question to ask when an objection or concern is raised).

Consent is only required for a hospital post-mortem, which is usually requested when the cause of death is not clear (e.g. the cause of illness was not evident during life) or for education or research purpose. Consent must be taken from the next of kin for this kind of post-mortem. According to the Human Tissue Act, it is an offence to remove, retain, or use human tissues, so a separate consent is required if any of this is intended. Relatives have the option of asking for a limited autopsy to be performed. For a coroner's post-mortem, however, consent is not required, and relatives cannot object to it, as it is a statutory process.

Some people may object to a post-mortem on religious grounds (e.g. Muslim, Jewish) or ask for the body to be released on the same day. It is not up to the medical registrar to make a decision regarding this in the middle of the night! Your job is only to tell the family why you must refer to the coroner and what will happen next. You can, however, reassure the family that the coroner will take their beliefs into consideration and discuss with them directly.

Coroners will never order a post-mortem examination without careful consideration and when there is the option of a non-invasive autopsy with computed tomography scan, which may reveal the cause of death in most cases. However, if required by law, a full post-mortem will have to be carried out (e.g. suspected foul play and the cause of death is not clear after a non-invasive autopsy).

He says there is no religious reason for his request; he just didn't want his wife's body to be mutilated.

- Gently tell him that *he cannot object to a coroner's post-mortem.*

  'The coroner and the pathologist will go through her medical notes and consider the facts very carefully. They'll take the decision to do a post-mortem only if it is absolutely necessary. I'm afraid we cannot object if the coroner decides to proceed with the post-mortem, as it is a legal process.'

He asks what exactly happens during a post-mortem and if that will definitely reveal the cause of her death.

- Briefly *explain the process of post-mortem examination* without going too much into the gory details.

  'Post-mortems are done by the pathologist, who will be assisted by qualified technicians. They will make an incision on the chest and tummy, remove the organs to study them, and then put them back. If they decide to retain the organs for further study, they will inform you. They will neatly close the wounds and dress the body, so even if you decide to use an open casket, no one will know that she has had a post-mortem. They'll take great care to ensure that the appearance of your wife is not altered.'

- Tell him that *the autopsy may or may not reveal the cause of her death.*

  'The post-mortem may or may not reveal the cause of her death. The coroner will decide the next steps if the post-mortem is unhelpful.'

He asks what will happen next.

- Tell him that the coroner will be informed.

  'We will now inform the police, who will take your wife's body to a special mortuary. They'll inform the coroner, who will then consult the pathologist and decide if a post-mortem is required. Please do not make any funeral arrangements until you hear from the coroner. He will let you know as soon as her body is ready to be released. Once the investigations are completed, the coroner will register the death, and you can get the death certificate.'

End the conversation by providing information on bereavement services. (*'I'll give you some information on bereavement services. They'll provide the necessary support to you and your family, which I am sure you will find immensely helpful during this very difficult time.'*)

SUMMARY

This scenario tests your skills in explaining the process of referral to the coroner for an unexplained death. You will be expected to:

- Demonstrate your understanding of (1) the situations in which you cannot complete an MCCD, (2) the process of referring to the coroner, and (3) the issues around performing a post-mortem examination.
- Sensitively communicate this to the bereaved husband, who is in a state of shock after losing his wife unexpectedly.

Before you walk into the room, the main challenge to anticipate is an objection from the husband for a post-mortem to be carried out or a request for the body to be released on the same day (usually for religious reasons). As it is a statutory process, giving them incorrect information or conveying false hopes (e.g. telling them that a post-mortem can be skipped if they do not consent) will result in an unsatisfactory mark for clinical communication, addressing concerns, and clinical judgement.

A variation of this scenario is to ask for consent from a relative to perform a hospital post-mortem for a patient who dies after a prolonged unexplained illness. You must (1) discuss the reasons for proposing a post-mortem (it may be important for families, too, to know the cause of death and get closure), (2) tell them that the knowledge gained from performing a post-mortem can be applied to similar cases in the future, (3) offer the option of a limited post-mortem, and (4) ask for permission to retain the organs should it be necessary.

Index

Printed in the United States
by Baker & Taylor Publisher Services